CREATIVE

D 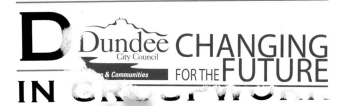 CHANGING FOR THE FUTURE

IN GROUPWORK

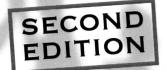

SECOND EDITION

Sue Jennings

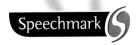

Speechmark Publishing Ltd
70 Alston Drive, Bradwell Abbey, Milton Keynes MK13 9HG, United Kingdom
www.speechmark.net

This book is dedicated with much love to my mother Alice Edna Jennings, a dancer and counsellor, who was a very creative person herself.

Published by **Speechmark Publishing Ltd**,

70 Alston Drive, Bradwell Abbey, Milton Keynes MK13 9HG, United Kingdom

Tel: +44 (0) 1908 326 944   Fax: +44 (0) 1908 326 960

www.speechmark.net

002-5675/Printed in the United Kingdom by CMP (UK) Ltd

British Library Cataloguing in Publication Data

A catalogue record for this book is available from the British Library

ISBN 978 0 86388 791 8

Contents

Preface to the Second Edition

Since this book was first published in 1986, much has changed
in the fields of therapies and work with people with special
needs. Language has changed, organisations have changed and
training and the 'professionalisation' of many activities has shifted
the whole landscape of this type of work. All the arts are now
accepted as 'Arts Therapies' and are State Registered with the
Health Professionals Council (HPC): dramatherapy, art therapy,
music therapy and soon dance-movement therapy. There is now
protection of title so that no one may call their work one of the
arts therapies or refer to themselves as an arts therapist unless
they have undertaken an approved course of training that leads
to a recognised qualification. These training courses are taught at
Masters level by universities (see Resources).

This means that we need to be careful of how we describe our
creative groupwork and I am pleased that I thought of this title
at the time. There is no legislation concerning creative drama in
groupwork, which is a practical approach but it is not therapy. It may
well be therapeutic and have a therapeutic effect on participants.

Overall, I am pleased to say that there is much more acceptance by
medical staff of the creative arts in the realms of 'mental ill-health'
and 'learning needs' and a greater understanding that it can have
a primary effect on people's brain development. Small children in
particular benefit from a creative playful relationship that will help
them develop resilience and confidence.

Many of these techniques can be adapted for work with children,
as I have always said – it is time to find the treasure!

New acknowledgements

I have many people to thank for stimulation, support and sources during the preparation of this book. At the beginning I must thank my PA Sue Hall for her constant attention and contributions to this manuscript.

I am very appreciative of my children and their spouses and grandchildren who have taught me such a lot about creativity and play.

Special dear friends including Åse Minde, Alida Gersie and Ann Cattanach, all the A people, have been supportive and stimulating in work and play.

My husband Peter is my dear friend and wonderful fun to be with.

Sue Jennings
Glastonbury 2010

Introduction to the Second Edition

Drama for all

Although many readers will be working in clinical settings such as hospitals, others will be involved in the increasing use of community rather than institutional care. There will also be those who work in the educational field. In all of these areas the working climate has been undergoing rapid and often drastic change. Both personnel and equipment are more scarce; and professionals must function as best they can in the context of limited resources.

This book reflects such changes and does not assume that resources are limitless. It is an optimistic book in that it aims to make things possible.

Drama can help all of us, if we choose to explore its potential. For example, it may enable us to acquire the clarity and conviction which we need in the debating group, the administration meeting or with management. It is intended that this book should reduce the historical gulf between 'us' and 'them', between the givers and the receivers, by acknowledging the potential in drama for ourselves and all the people with whom we work.

A book is no substitute for training and experience, particularly in a dynamic medium such as creative drama. Therefore, the reader is urged to take courage and experiment, to seek advice (and, of course, supervision), and to learn by 'reflective action'. It is *not* advisable simply to use these pages as a working manual.

How to use this book

Part I of this book should be read in its entirety before selecting material from Part II. What has been attempted is to provide pointers, to draw attention to issues which may not yet have been addressed by people intending to practise, to share some of the author's considerable accumulated knowledge of the subject, and to stimulate the reader's own innate creativity. The guidelines given in the following chapters will encourage users to try things for themselves and take some risks, so that new ideas and techniques may emerge.

The exercises listed in Part 2 will undoubtedly provide the basis for many group sessions. However, group leaders should discuss and plan and generate their own variations on exercises and games. Above all, there is much to be gained from careful thought before each session, and by reflection during and after the event. Guidance on how to use the exercises in Part 2 can be found on page 33.

A word of encouragement

This book has been written because I believe that everybody is potentially creative, whether worker or client. Some of us have to discover or rediscover our own creativity; and some of us are tired or jaded. Others are daunted when faced with groups that are too large, with clients who have multiple needs and with constantly diminishing resources.

Working with this book won't change your budget. However, it could give you some new energy and sense of worth so that you go on with inspiration.

Remember that creativity is catching. If you can feel creative and spontaneous and above all hopeful, the people you work with will also experience these feelings.

Creative drama is an adventure and, like all adventures, has inherent risks and dangers. Nevertheless it can also be playful, enriching – and sometimes magic.

Go slay the dragon and bring back the treasures!

Sue Jennings

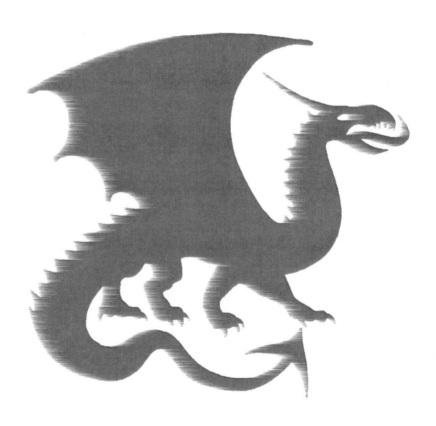

Introduction

A significant proportion of readers of this book will be professionals who are already familiar with running groups of various kinds. Others may have used drama-related activities such as role play with clients in their own field of work. There may also be those who would very much like to venture into the use of drama, but who have as yet lacked the courage to try it.

Many features of groupwork such as group dynamics are broadly similar, no matter what the setting, and it is not proposed to discuss general issues here. However, a creative drama group may differ in certain respects from other therapeutic or social skills groups; and it is the distinctive nature, scope and underlying philosophy of such work that will be considered in this opening chapter. Drama has been used for the purposes of healing, education, spiritual enlightenment and ritual for many centuries in the Western world (viz. early Greek theatre). In other cultures ritual still plays a most important role.

Specific application of therapy through the medium of drama began to take shape in the early 1960s, when mime, movement and improvisation were found to produce encouraging results with groups of people with learning needs and people with mental ill-health. The approaches adopted were so favourably received that nurses, therapists, psychologists, psychiatrists and social workers became increasingly interested in the potentialities of drama. Teachers have also explored drama within education, in particular special education, with comparable success, for example, among low achievers. Two fields of work have now emerged, namely Social Theatre and Dramatherapy, each generating new ideas and research. The rationale of this book and the ideas put forward derive from many years of practical experience in both these fields.

The reader who is relatively unfamiliar with these activities may wish to refer to the Bibliography. It is hoped that the increasing number of dramatherapists will also find value in this book. Although it is not written for a specific profession, emphasis is placed on *good practice*, which in turn should be the aim of any worker using creative drama with groups. While the author would like to see trained dramatherapists working alongside other professionals in a whole range of settings, such an ideal situation is still relatively rare. Furthermore, the application of drama in groupwork spreads beyond the remit of a single profession. Many share the philosophy that 'doing' (ie action) is an important way of bringing about change. Sadly, we tend to divide people into the doers and the thinkers. This book, however, is about doing *and* thinking, or 'reflective action'. It is intended to circumvent the professional boundaries of different disciplines and to refer to areas which are of common concern to all who work with people.

Why drama?

In the past, the use of drama in groupwork has either been considered too 'dangerous', and therefore to be avoided at all costs, or else it has been used as a Friday afternoon filler when nothing in particular has been planned. A variation on the latter is the 'Drama is good for you' approach, in which such activities have been used almost as one might prescribe a daily dose of laxative. There exists some notion that drama will do you good but no one stops to ask the question – why? In the following sections there will be an opportunity to ask such questions in order to refine our practice and be selective in its applications.

Creative drama is intrinsic to human development as we can observe in the early reactions between mothers and their newborn children (Jennings, 2009). We imitate expressions within hours of being born and continue to 'dramatise' our situation through dramatic play.

However, drama also needs to be understood alongside theatre where we can see stories and plays that touch our souls. Live theatre cannot be superseded by films or television. The human interaction that can happen between audience and performers can bring about insight and change in ways that often surprise us!

Empathy and security

Whatever the context or composition of the group, two factors will always apply. First, while training in this work increases confidence and improves the range of skills, a leader's attitude and ability to empathise are always of paramount importance.

Second, a well run group has, by its very nature, great therapeutic potential: within it, members can find a sense of community, security and support. Here, they may explore, take risks, increase their understanding of self, build confidence and also make changes. Creative drama in a group setting can be a means of finding out about the unknown whilst, at the same time, having an equal value in reinforcing the known.

About the author

Sue Jennings grew up as a dancer and actress before developing a strong interest in drama and theatre as therapy. She has been working in this field for over 50 years and she has established training courses in the UK, Romania, Czech Republic and Greece. She studied postgraduate social anthropology at the London School of Economics and School of Oriental and African Studies (University of London) and completed her doctoral research with the Temiar peoples of Malaysia (published by Routledge as *Theatre, Ritual and Transformation: The Senoi Temiars*, 1994).

Sue has written more than 25 books, seven of them with Speechmark. Sue still works as a trainer and supervisor and conducts play therapy and dramatherapy consultations.

Sue and her partner Peter live and work in Glastonbury and Romania where they lead projects for people with special needs.

To contact Sue:
sue@rowancentre.net and suejphd@gmail.com

For more information on courses, projects and publications
www.suejennings.com   www.dramatherapy.net
www.projectwolf.co.uk   www.rowancentre.net

Part 1
The Scope & Possibilities of Creative Drama in Groupwork

1 Exploration of Structure and Roles in Group Drama

Structure

Social psychologists have observed that we organise our lives in a dramatic structure or framework. We can view ourselves and others in a series of scenes and episodes, some of which have a consciously predictable structure, such as when we organise a celebration or a formal meeting. Such scenes have a conscious 'test' and usually the 'roles' are prescribed. Each scene has its 'key actors', a 'supporting cast', and a known ending.

There are other scenes which do not appear to be predictable – chance meetings; informal gatherings; daily interactions with the family. However, on examination we find that many of these scenes can have predictable elements including an unacknowledged 'sub-text', 'roles' which may be inflexible, and a seemingly inevitable ending.

During the course of certain creative drama exercises, a formal and less formal structure of interaction can be explored by members of the group.

Embodiment-Projection-Role (EPR)

EPR is a very useful developmental structure that can be used with any type of group and ensures that you follow a developmental progression in the groupwork. EPR follows the same developmental sequence that takes place in child development from birth to 7 years. The first 12 months of a baby's life is mainly physical and sensory (Embodiment); everything is experienced through the body, whether it is large movements or tiny eyelash flutters. Sensory and dramatic play between mothers and babies form the healthy core of the attachment relationship. Around 13 months the infant becomes more interested in the world beyond the body in terms of objects and substances (toys, sand and water, messy play), progressing to puzzle play, drawing and painting, doll and puppet play; all forms of projective play (P). At around 3–4 years old we can observe that children start to go back into themselves again and instead of projecting roles and stories through the puppets, they play the roles (R) themselves (see Bibliography for further information). This brief illustration shows the importance in the sequencing of Embodiment-Projection-Role and how we can use this sequence to structure our sessions: starting with movement and physical warm-ups, then moving on to drawing and painting and then to playing roles.

Roles

There is sometimes a reluctance to admit that we constantly engage in role playing. It is the word 'playing', perhaps, that makes us feel it is not *real*. Or is it that being in a role somehow implies that we are not being ourselves?

In fact, each one of us adopts a variety of roles; indeed, it is important to remember that we develop the capacity to role play from a very early age – about ten months. It is most significant that we become, as it were, 'mobile in character', even before we become 'mobile in body'. Our role play is further developed through play in childhood and through experimentation in adolescence, whilst also being shaped by the family and outside world. On reaching adulthood, each individual has embraced a variety of roles which together form our role repertoire, by means of which our external and internal worlds are related.

In creative drama groups, individuals may be found to have difficulty in making connections between these internal and external facets.

Others may have developed rigid and fixed roles in early life; or else inappropriate roles have emerged, often through inadequate or faulty 'modelling'. Drama not only helps us come to terms with our everyday life and facilitates exploration of our inner life, but it also enables us to transcend ourselves and go beyond our everyday limits and boundaries.

Through various forms of dramatic structure and dramatic role play the group leader aims to help group members achieve some of the following:

- *expand* the limits of their experience and stimulate their artistic and aesthetic sense

- *uncover* the predictable structures that trap people in unhelpful behaviours and find some creative alternatives

- *redevelop* appropriate roles through practice and remodelling until they become more natural and less conscious

- *encourage* the extension of role repertoire, ie, a range of roles that are appropriate to different situations

- *create* new possibilities for experiencing scenes in unusual or unprescribed ways

- *discover* ways of connecting internalised responses with external behaviour, and vice versa.

The basic premise for the above section is that we all have potential for some change – of life, of love, of vision – given the opportunity and the right kind of support. One way in which to explore these possibilities is through drama, for which *everyone* has potential – although they may not be aware of it.

2 The Focus of Drama Work in Groups

Those who venture into drama work with groups naturally hope that their approach will produce creative results and encourage expression, while also perhaps bringing about new insights and enabling members to accomplish tasks. However, as described in 'Models of Practice in Dramatherapy' (Jennings, 1983), a specific focus tends to emerge, largely determined by the type and needs of the group members. Three fairly distinct types of focus can be identified. These are described below and form the basis for advice offered in later sections. The exercises in Part II have also been classified according to these categories although many of the activities can be used to achieve different objectives simply by presenting them in a different way, thus making them suitable for more than one of the following types of group.

Focus on Creativity and Expression

The emphasis in such a group is placed on the creative development and aesthetic experience of the participants. Drama activities can include movement, mime and improvisation; puppets and masks; and text and story work. Members may also be encouraged to focus on performance, such as seasonal celebrations. Productions should avoid becoming competitive, but it is sometimes valuable for creative experiences to be shared with a wider audience.

Apart from giving creative and aesthetic enjoyment, a group of this nature provides stimulation, encouragement and a heightened experience of self. The work also increases an individual's confidence through development of the imagination and the tapping of undiscovered potential. Furthermore, it improves communication and encourages cooperation (an important social skill), for members have to work together to create an improvisation or production. The leader's role as facilitator is most important: a balance has to be struck between allowing the group's creative energies to meander without any sort of direction, and imposing the leader's own opinions and ideas as to how the activity should develop.

Creative drama groups have potential with many sorts of people, whatever their age and circumstances.

Focus on Tasks, Skills and Learning

In a group of this nature, the behaviour and skills of everyday life can be rehearsed and refined or modified through the medium of drama in a variety of activities such as role play. Some skills develop as a by-product of creative drama work; other programmes must be specifically designed. Skills acquired may include simple communication or training in the use of non-verbal signs; initiating conversation; or improving conceptual skills like problem solving. Group members can gain experience of decision making and negotiation, and begin to develop some autonomy as well as cooperative skills. This drama work is very goal specific; and it is often developed, for example, in rehabilitation groups in prisons, psychiatric hospitals and children's homes.

The work planned for a group with a focus on 'skills' is likely to form one part of an overall programme of training or education; and in such a group, the leader's role as 'model' is especially important.

Focus on Insight, Self Awareness and Change

Here, the focus is again entirely different. An 'insight-type' group would be set up for the benefit of particular clients such as acute admissions groups and those people in family and marital therapy (or indeed all those groups already mentioned).

Within the context of the group, unconscious processes may be given creative expression by enacting scenes from past, present and future, and sometimes by recreating the themes of dreams and fantasies. The drama activities selected for work of this kind give members an opportunity to explore their own feelings and relationships within the security of the group.

All the work on role play and media skills which may be used by the 'creative' drama group may also be used here. However, it is understood in an 'insight' group that self discovery and change are the aims and that, for this purpose, the group represents 'life', the family or the outside world. Members are encouraged to reflect on their own experiences, and the group also becomes the scenario within which possible changes can be explored. By use of symbolism, certain mental or physical blocks may be resolved through new insights and increased confidence.

The leader will be likely to run such a group as a 'closed' group, namely to make it available only to the original membership who should remain constant in the relatively long term. Depending upon the degree of experience of the leader and the rationale of the group, 'interpretation of experiences' may not be emphasised. Often, gradually emerging conscious awareness of previously unacknowledged difficulties, *without* the use of verbal analysis or interpretation, proves to be of greatest value.

3 Before Setting up a Group

Rationale and Objectives

Before embarking on the detailed planning which is involved in setting up any group activity, it is as well to give careful thought to the rationale of a potential drama group, and to administrative considerations. The following questions are intended to alert the reader to possible pitfalls and to help in ascertaining the leader's main objectives.

Why?	
Why start a group in the first place?	Has a need been established? Are the staff skills available? Are there suitable clients?
Why choose drama rather than other skills or creative processes?	Are there specific or general goals? Is the work experimental? Research? Is drama the main focus for therapy? Or is it a support therapy?

What?	
What model of group will it be?	Will it be open to new members? Will it be a closed group from the outset?
What emphasis will the group have?	Will it focus on creativity, tasks or insight?
What numbers are planned?	Will there be a fixed number? Should a minimum or maximum number be set? (10 is a good size for a group: people with profound learning difficulties need smaller groups.)

What staff ratio is planned?	Will there be a single leader? Will there be a co-leader? Will there be assistants/students?
What will be the role of assistants/students in relation to the clients?	Should they interact in the group in the same way as clients? Will they act purely as assistants to the leader?
What will be the duration of the group?	Will it span 10 weeks; 20 weeks; a year? (If possible, avoid open-ended arrangements.)
What will be the frequency and length of sessions?	1 hour twice a week? 1½ hours once a week? (See Planning and Preparation pp16–21)
What sort of records will be kept of individuals or group activities?	Will these be formal or informal? Will video or written notes be used? Confidentiality? Data protection? Remember to record and monitor *your* feelings and processes.

How?

How will members be recruited to the group?	By self-referral?
How will people know about the group?	By publicity or a talk? Via the referring agent? Via a notice board or announcement?
How will people be selected for the group	Open to all comers? By interview? By medical or other selection?
How will aims and goals be established?	Will they be fixed by the leader? Will they be negotiable?

How?	
How will this group relate to the overall programme?	Will it be unconnected? Will it be an integral part of a programme? Will it be a choice with other activities?
How will breaks for illness or holidays be covered?	Natural breaks? Substitute leader available? Co-leader available?

Where?	
Where will the group be held?	Are you responsible for a space? Must space be negotiated? Is there a suitable space?
Where are the emergency facilities?	Where is the First Aid Box? Where is the spare key? Where is the Fire Extinguisher/Fire Escape?
Where will the leader find support?	Are colleagues available? Can friends provide support?

Who?	
Who will provide supervision?	Will this come from outside? Will the institution provide it? Will it be individual or in a group setting?
Who is responsible for the management and organisation of the group?	The institution? The team? The leader?
Who coordinates the overall treatment programme?	The institution? The team? The leader?

Clarifying Aims

Whilst considering what type and focus of group is required, and having worked through administrative and other details, it is also advisable for the leader to be clear about the overall aims for the group. It has been found from experience that conflicts can arise if the aims of the institution and the group members are not compatible with those of the leader.

The following simple chart has been devised to assist in identifying potential areas of dissonance *before* the group is set up. The reader may wish to redesign the chart or the headings.

Clarifying Aims	
A My aims for the group	**B** The institution's aims for the group
C The group's aims for themselves	**D** My aims for myself

Sample of how the above chart has been used in practice:

A	B
1 Provide a structure for change 2 Develop trust and cooperation 3 Develop communication	1 Keep group meaningfully busy 2 Avoid confrontation; keep atmosphere calm 3 Maintain status quo
C	**D**
1 Relieve boredom 2 Feel better 3 Sleep properly	1 Develop work professionally 2 Feel satisfaction at achieving aims 3 Develop myself

The reader is invited to consider the above chart where we see that the aims of A and C are not wholly incompatible. The aims of A and B, however, might give rise to conflict (viz. A1 in direct opposition to B3). The leader can reflect on how, for example, D3 can be achieved and whether the potential difficulties identified could be avoided.

It is always important to discuss the aims of the group with group members, and it may be that further discussion is needed in subsequent sessions.

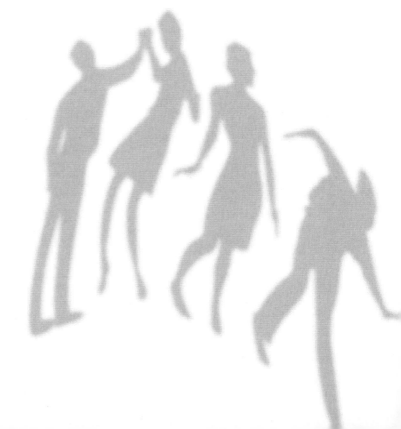

4 Supervision and Training

Supervision and Support

As previously mentioned, to achieve the best results in creative drama, regular supervision is essential. Because of the nature of this work, a leader may tend towards over-involvement, excessive use of energy, and a counter-productive degree of identification with members of the group. Supervision, by providing support and feedback, helps keep all the processes moving forwards and enables the leader to discuss details, to plan ahead and to function with the right degree of compassionate detachment.

Supervision should be provided by an experienced person, preferably a senior working colleague and it may have to be sought if it does not exist.

Support networks may be both professional and social and are also very important. The leader of a group should be sure to make regular opportunities for 'switching off' from work. A more balanced outlook on the activities of a group and on work in general can be achieved if there are creative or other activities to occupy one's leisure time.

Training

If any professional worker is interested in pursuing creative drama work with groups, some specific training is warmly recommended. Training courses, whilst limited in their locations, are increasing in number. Those who have already taken a dramatherapy course are encouraged to attend for further training in order to extend their range of skills. Courses of varying length are listed in the Resources.

5 Some Words of Caution

When running a creative drama group we must bear in mind that all therapeutic work can occasionally stimulate unexpected reactions to particular techniques. Drama is no exception; indeed it may give rise to some unhelpful results in certain circumstances.

Whilst it is not realistic to hope to cover every contingency in a book of this size, some essential basic guidelines are given below. The reader is reminded that it is always advisable to obtain regular supervision and that advice should be sought if a leader is in any doubt about an activity or the behaviour of an individual group member.

General Advice

- Guard against thinking of drama simply as a collection of techniques. Remember it is a *creative process* which can tap experience at a very profound level.

- *Never* introduce a new idea or activity to a group without having tried it out. Always experiment first on yourself and colleagues.

- Develop 'antennae' and be sensitive to the group's changing needs and moods. Members will often know 'where they need to go' and what they are ready for, even if they cannot yet verbalise it.

- Aim to act as a catalyst rather than a controller. Be alert to this situation and avoid using phrases such as 'We've *got* to do this'; 'I'll *make* them do that' or 'They *have* to ....'

Situations to Handle with Special Care

- Highly stimulating material is not appropriate for severely anxious or hyperactive groups.

- When initiating role play remember that to 'be someone else' can be a very disturbing experience for people who are not comfortable in their own identity.

- Appearing to 'get lost in an activity' is not necessarily an indication of fruitful involvement.

- An apparently 'cathartic' group experience is not always an indication of a 'good' session. And the evidence of catharsis is not necessarily a highly visible expression of emotion.

- Direct techniques can be unhelpful for some people because the end product may be perceived as reinforcing the unsatisfactory present rather than pointing to a hopeful future.

6 Planning and Preparation

It is a mistake to imagine that what may appear to be an informal, unstructured, creative drama session needs no pre-planned framework. The most successful sessions are those which have a beginning, a middle and an end; which are kept to a pre-arranged time; and in which the leader maintains an imperceptible yet confident 'steadying hand' on the way group activities evolve.

When planning for creative drama work, a leader should first endeavour to find a suitable setting for the group. This need not be luxurious. In fact carpets, for example, are a handicap. However, it is helpful to have sufficient space, light and some fresh air. A wooden or cork tile floor is ideal; and rostra are preferable to either upright chairs or floor cushions because they are more flexible. Good lighting is also an asset.

Preparation for drama sessions requires considerable forethought. It is necessary to decide upon an overall framework for work with the group so that it develops sequentially and ideas are linked from session to session.

The great advantage of structure is that, within it, there can be flexibility. Each group is like a living, growing organism which responds to its members and its leader who are also living, changing organisms. A leader develops the capacity to respond to the needs and mood of the group through his or her own spontaneity and creativity. Initially, the inexperienced will rely heavily on detailed planning of each session. However, in time and with practice, this structure can be allowed greater flexibility as the leader puts increasing trust in intuition and judgement.

The following diagram illustrates how a session can be planned. The ideal session length for a group of 10 clients is 1½ hours. Within this span adequate time must be allowed for warming-up or 'opening' activities, for 'development' which involves the main work of the session, and for a satisfactory and relaxed winding-up or 'closure'.

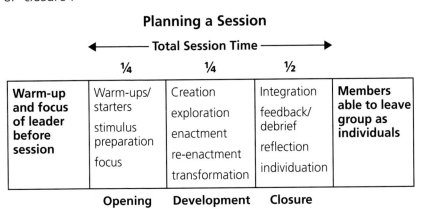

Planning a Session

←———— Total Session Time ————→

	¼	¼	½	
Warm-up and focus of leader before session	Warm-ups/ starters stimulus preparation focus	Creation exploration enactment re-enactment transformation	Integration feedback/ debrief reflection individuation	**Members able to leave group as individuals**
	Opening	**Development**	**Closure**	

Even before the session begins, the leader must make time to warm-up and 'focus', in other words to get emotionally and mentally prepared for action.

Vitality and a sense of purpose must be conveyed to the group when they first arrive. They should be greeted with an air of warmth and confidence, for some may be feeling nervous, anxious or even antagonistic. Time should not be wasted before embarking on the appropriate warm-up or starter activities such as are described in Part II. This opening phase, which should last not more than one quarter of the total session, involves stimulation and preparation for the development phase, and begins to focus attention on the area of work to be covered.

The development phase should span not more than half of the total session time. Within the space of perhaps 45 minutes, the group may be active in creating a story, mask or scene; in exploring feelings, a theme or a topic (perhaps through improvisation); in either exploratory or goal-specific role play (*enactment*); or in re-enacting an experience which may be either invented or real, myth or fantasy.

The leader will have selected games or other activities through which some, but by no means all, of the above can be developed. For some groups or in some sessions, this will be a time for exploring and working on change in members' feelings (*transformation*).

For the final quarter of the session, more restful exercises are chosen through which the group can make a gradual transition from the focus of the session back to the focus of everyday activities. Material and feelings which have been put in focus must now be 're-owned' (*integration*). New insights are absorbed and group members are encouraged to reflect on what has taken place rather than only to rely on feedback from others (*reflection*). These two processes may not necessarily occur within a group session but time and space must nonetheless be provided for that possibility.

Techniques of distancing and relaxing may be employed in order to help members reconstrue themselves as separate individuals who relate to, but are not fused with, the group (*individuation*).

Finally, when the session is brought to a close (*on time*, and gently but firmly), each member should be in a frame of mind which enables him or her to leave as an individual in a relaxed manner. After the session, a leader should make some notes on what took place, what exercises were used, and what reactions they produced. Leaders should also learn to monitor their own reactions and bodily feelings, and record the 'process' of the group, as well as recording the feedback from the group.

Sample Sessions

The following sample sessions suggest how a group session may be 'thought through', with different exercises being selected according to needs. They also show how the same techniques may be used to respond to different needs.

It should be stressed that the three examples offer no more than guidelines and should not therefore be interpreted as set formulae.

• Example 1
Creative expressive focus
Residential setting for elderly people
Duration of session: 1 hour
Grouping: 6–8 people.

Aims and objectives	To counteract institutionalisation; to provide a physical stimulus; to emphasise identity; to reinforce simple choices; and to encourage creativity.
Warm-up phase	**Physical:** Starter exercises 2, 3, 4 (p35) for example (you may wish to use a CD for rhythmic movement – what we call 'Easy Listening' – rather than anything too loud or fast). **Names:** Starter exercises 16, 17, 18 (on p37) for example.
Development phase	Exercises selected will depend on how familiar the group is with drama activities. The above exercises may be sufficient during early sessions; closing with a quiet relaxation activity such as 2.1, 2.2, 2.3 (pp52–54). Otherwise continue with basic storytelling ideas such as 6.1, 6.2, 6.3 (pp140–142). People always enjoy the opportunity to tell stories whether it is their own story or a story from the radio, television or newspaper. Make sure that everyone has a turn.
Closure phase	Relaxation such as 16 or 17 under and Cool Downs and Closures (p171) or a relaxation exercise such as 2.1, 2.2, 2.3 (pp52–54).

- **Example 2**
Task centred focus
Rehabilitation group for prisoners
Duration of session: 1½ hours
Grouping: 10 people

Aims and objectives	To develop flexibility in dealing with various situations; to prepare for return to life 'outside'; to experience managing rather than being managed; and to develop trust and communication skills.
Warm-up phase	**Physical:** A selection of different games from the Warm-ups and Starter section (see pp35–50) will encourage group members to collaborate both with the whole group as well as in pairs. It will depend on whether the individuals have had previous drama experience as to the pace of the preparation of the Warm-up phase.
	Voice: Many individuals need support to 'find their voice' and to use it appropriately so try exercises from the Warm-ups and Starter section such as 52 and 56 (on pp41–42).
Development phase	Goal-specific role play that can explore future situations is appropriate for this group. For example 5.8 'Sculpts and Everyday Life' (see p125) can be used to focus the group and then invite the group to suggest scenes and situations that they feel would be difficult to handle.
Closure phase	Allow members of the group to discuss how they felt during the exercises and to consider whether comparisons can be drawn with feelings they have experienced before. You could finish the group with 16 or 17 from the Cool Downs and Closures section (see p171).

- **Example 3**
Insight and personal development
Children with emotional and behavioural needs
Duration of session: 1 hour
Grouping: 6 people.

Aims and objectives	To develop awareness whilst taking into account hostility towards families which may not have been verbalised; to limit work to the one-hour session, since anxiety levels may be high; and to increase members' trust in their peers and their leader.
Warm-up phase	**Games:** Encourage the energy in the group by using basic games such as 63, 64, 65 on p43 and encourage everyone to literally warm-up (any exercises on pp35–36 from nos. 1–15).
	Names: Develop awareness of each other through exercises 17 and 19 (p37).
	Feelings: Introduce expression with exercises 95 and 96 (p47).
Development phase	Children can free play with toys and puppets and then focus on a family story about the animal or puppets. Stories can be shared with the group, still keeping within the metaphor of the toys. This allows the children to play safely without feeling exposed.
Closure phase	Discuss with the children any difficulties they think the animals might be having and what could be done about it. Invite the group members to put away the toys and puppets as 'ordinary toys' and not as characters in the stories.

7 Equipment

Things to Acquire

Creative drama requires little in the way of elaborate props or expensive equipment. However, a sturdy CD player (which has the right adaptor and someone who knows how to work it!) is a valuable asset. A selection of CDs should be carefully chosen for appropriate movement and relaxation exercises. In addition, it is helpful to have a supply of large sheets of paper, a quantity of felt tip pens, an unlimited supply of newspapers and some large cardboard boxes. For role play exercises it may be appropriate to accumulate a general 'dressing up' collection including a wide variety of hats and caps and perhaps some chiffon strips and scarves.

A range of toys, zoo and farm animals and a box of miscellaneous small objects can be used in creating spectrograms and pictograms; and stiff card and some craft materials would be needed if the group were working with masks.

For further equipment suggestions, look at *Drama and Play with Adults at Risk* (Jennings, 2005b).

Things to Make

Puppets and masks should, wherever possible, be made with the group and not *for* them. This may, however, be impractical for people with severe needs.

Simple role play cards, to accompany some of the exercises described in Part II, can be made very easily by using small library cards which are convenient to store. Print in large and clear letters with a dark felt pen, putting one phrase on each card. For example, write a stimulating opening line on each card: 'We had just settled down for tea when there was a knock at the door'.

Simpler cards can be prepared for those who are not ready for full role play exercises. In this case, elements of a role can be identified and a variety of feelings, for example, can be written on separate cards. When each member has taken a card, individuals may be asked to imagine, 'How do I *sit* with this feeling?' or 'How do I *look* with this feeling?' (An example of this type of activity can be found in Part 2, 98–100, p48).

Pair cards are versatile additions to basic resources. Using these, characters may be asked to 'find' each other in a game or role play (eg mother/father/baby; farmer/cow; master/slave). Apropos of the latter type of activity, male/female options should be kept open and stereotypes avoided wherever possible. Pair cards can also be used when comparing and contrasting feelings such as happy/sad, or when looking at qualities and characteristics in improvisations (eg 'I like to be in charge' / 'I like to be told what to do').

8 Negotiating a Contract

At the first official session, although individuals may have been previously interviewed and the general purpose of the group discussed, the leader should spend perhaps half of the time developing a rapport with the group, giving necessary information and agreeing a contract with the members. This contract should encompass what is expected of the group but should also take into account what the leader has to offer to them.

A positive working alliance must be established between the group and its leader in this first session; and this can be achieved by discussing and agreeing on its direction and specific aims. In the absence of such an alliance, cooperation from individual members cannot be guaranteed. Experience has shown that negative feelings may later be transferred to the leader, or certain group members may resort to 'acting out'. Naturally, the level of discussion and the flexibility of the contract must depend upon the type of setting and the nature of the clients. If the verbal skills of the group are limited, it may be helpful to use 'action method' to work out the contract (eg role play illustrating punctuality or confidentiality). If this is the case, then a smooth transition must be achieved between this introductory activity and the rest of the session.

Many operational details need to be agreed and the leader is advised to prepare a mental list of matters to raise informally with the group. A list of possible issues for consideration is provided below. This is intended purely as a guideline.

Points to Raise and Discuss with the Group

1   What are the aims and intentions of the group? **(Goals)**

2   How will the group achieve those aims? **(Methods)**

3   What skills and experience has the leader got that could be beneficial to the group and vice versa? **(Expectations)**

4   What does it mean to have an 'open/closed' group? **(Framework)**

5   If it is a closed group, how are leaving and entry to be agreed? **(Negotiation)**

6   Does 'anything go' or are there limits on behaviour, eg aggression? **(Boundaries)**

7   What should be the starting and finishing times? **(Punctuality)**

8   What is agreed about smoking/refreshments, etc? **(Ground rules)**

9   What happens to personal information/photographs? **(Confidentiality)**

10 How will ground rules and limits be maintained? **(Consensus)**

9 Opening a Session

Having given careful thought to various aspects of the group, as outlined in earlier sections, and having planned an appropriate mix of activities for the current session, one final piece of preparation is advised. In order to gain members' interest and cooperation from the moment they arrive, the leader needs to make mental preparation beforehand. For, just as a 'cold' group tends to be unresponsive until it is 'warmed up', so the leader must warm up too. This is achieved by allowing sufficient time to think about the group, to re-read notes from the previous session, to consider what was achieved and to identify other themes which may be appropriate to explore. All other preoccupations should be put to one side while a group is in progress.

On the arrival of participants, a short time generally needs to be spent on 'starter' or 'warm-up' activities. These may serve as a preparation for the main business of the session, in which case the tone and type of exercises chosen will need to be compatible with the main focus. Warm-ups may also be used as an initial focus for members, particularly if the group arrives already warmed up but with animation and energy which would benefit from being channelled into some kind of structure.

Depending upon the nature and mood of the group, these introductory exercises may be used for warming up voices, reactions or general creativity; or they may serve as 'getting to know you' activities. When used in this way they might be described as providing a stimulus for the group.

Once the session is under way, the leader should 'listen' to the group's verbal and non-verbal messages, assessing their mood and noticing their reactions to activities, to the leader and to each other. Themes, too, may emerge naturally and can be incorporated into the work of the session by a perceptive leader.

If the current mood of the group is, for example, wary, then warm-ups may be used either to work with that mood or to dispel it, *or* to explore it. Likewise, fearful, 'tight' or anticipatory moods can be worked into the framework of the session if the leader remains responsive to the needs of the group. On occasion, a high level of anxiety may be noted at the beginning of a session, and some work on breathing and relaxation may be chosen to occupy the warm-up phase.

As a general rule, starters should be consistent with the overall strategy. Therefore, if a quiet reflective atmosphere is required because the development phase is to be spent creating sculpts, noisy or very physical warm-ups would naturally be inappropriate. If the whole group, small group or paired work is planned, then warm-ups can lay the foundations for this.

A word of advice in relation to the latter: do not make the mistake of asking a group to form pairs when there is an uneven number of participants! If pairs are essential then solve the dilemma by offering to be someone's partner first.

Warm-ups or opening exercises are described in Part II, under the following headings: to warm, names, breathing, voice, games, feelings, roles. The reader is advised to select one or two according to the various criteria discussed above, and bearing in mind the type of group, number of members, overall programme of work and current needs.

10 Developing a Session

Once a group has been warmed up and is beginning to focus on a theme, a task or an issue, the leader may use a range of methods to develop the session. This middle phase should not occupy more than half of the total session time.

In choosing activities, the leader not only takes into account whether the group is focusing on creativity, tasks or insight but should also consider 'where the group is at'. For example, a warm-up may have produced an unexpected result – an exercise may have been too difficult, leaving the group feeling somewhat inadequate (de-skilled). In this situation, it would be necessary to shift focus slightly and to build up group confidence again by re-working that warm-up in a different way.

The group may have arrived with 'left over business' from another situation or from the previous week's session. That, too, might require attention – perhaps in the development phase. If, however, the group appears ready to proceed, then activities may be structured in one of the following ways.

Creativity and Expression

When stimulating creativity, themes such as 'the sea' may be explored through movement; they may be dramatised through an improvisation; or they may be created in a drama or a text (eg *Sea Fever* by John Masefield). Finally, they may be refined through a performance.

Tasks and Skills

Working towards specific goals such as the achievement of listening or 'looking' skills, tasks may be practised in very small steps, eg gradually encouraging eye contact in someone who finds it extremely difficult. Example: the I-Spy game involves both listening and looking. Alternatively, they may be structured within a game (for example, Warm-ups and Starters 82 and 83 on pp45–46) or rehearsed through simulation, by re-creation of the real life situation.

Focus on Insight. Self Awareness and Change

In this type of group, participants will gradually lead where they wish the group to go. There is encouragement of the use of metaphors and symbols, and group members begin to work at a deeper level of meaning. Nevertheless a structure is important to safely contain the group and enable 'de-roling' and preparation for closure.

Summary

I have described a wealth of techniques that can be adapted and applied with most groups of people with special needs. There is a description of questions to be addressed before group work can start effectively on pp8–10 and 25.

There are over 100 warm-ups to start your groups and 'get them going' as well as closures in order to finish your groups' work in a calm manner. The warm-ups involve movement and dance, games and stories, preparation for role plays, breathing and relaxation. Movement and relaxation techniques slowly build up people's awareness and body image. There are plenty of games to build confidence and stimulate group interaction and cooperation.

Pictures and images allow people to develop their projective communication and creativity. There are careful descriptions of drama and role play that can address both real life and social skills as well as imaginative scenes to encourage development of the right brain hemisphere. There are yet more exercises for storytelling, puppets and masks.

When planning your groups try to keep to a 'through line' – so that everything is connected and not just a bunch of exercises applied at random. Try to try out your techniques on colleagues and friends before applying them for real.

If you are anxious there is a possibility that you may feel you should do lots of exercises. This means that there will be no time for assimilation of new ideas and insights. Remember that a lot of group work is fun and that it is fine for you to have fun too!

11 Closing a Session

A leader must learn to sense the appropriate moment at which to start 'closing' a session. It is ill-advised to over-run the planned time and then to say, three minutes before the end 'It's time for us to stop'. However, beware of interrupting a valuable piece of work that is proving very absorbing or intense, simply to impose an ending of the session. It is the leader's responsibility to bring about a 'de-climax', gradually working towards the closure. If members are deeply involved in an activity they should be brought slowly 'to the surface'. For example, if people are engaged in improvisation, they should be warned in good time, 'You have five minutes more, then we shall present this work to the other group members'.

During effective closure exercises, each individual de-intensifies the experience of the session. This may in some instances be achieved through gentle relaxation. Members should be encouraged to integrate their experiences through reflection. Reflection may often encompass their 'life as a whole' and not simply the experience of that session.

Any involvement in role play *must* include a 'de-roling' process whereby individuals acknowledge that they are 'themselves' again. Group members usually wish to share their experiences and may also give feedback to others. This should not, however, feel like an obligation. Each participant should be able to leave the group feeling he or she has a separate identity from other group members. This is what is described on page 18 as individuation, and involves facilitation of distancing and leaving.

Part 2
Practical Techniques

1 Warm-ups and Starters

Just as athletes need to warm up physically and we all need to 'streeetch' before doing a workout, everyone needs some kind of warm-up both to energise their bodies and to focus their minds. This preparation at the beginning will ensure that there are greater opportunities for creativity during your groupwork session.
The following 115 techniques take into account people who are not mobile and who may be sitting in chairs. You can use any combination of the following techniques:

Warm-ups and Starters

Warm-ups to warm 1 – 15

Warm-ups with names 16 – 30

Warm-ups with breathing 31 – 45

Warm-ups with voice 46 – 60

Warm-ups with games 61 – 90

Warm-ups with feelings 90 – 91

Warm-ups with roles 107 – 115

When choosing a warm-up remember that you will link it to the activity to follow. For example, if you are going to explore feelings, then you will choose a warm-up that focuses on feelings. However, everyone benefits from a general warm-up that includes both physical and vocal exercises. Whatever the exercise you will obviously modify them to suit the needs or abilities of your groups.

Warm-ups to WARM!

People need to be able to stretch their limbs, yawn and generally free their bodies for movement. Many people who live in institutions and elderly people spend a long time sitting and may need longer to 'get going'.

Invite the group to do the following activities:

1   Stand in a circle and first of all rub your hands together, then rub each arm from the shoulder to the wrist, especially the elbows. Rub your tummy using alternate hands making circles, rub your knees and then the backs of your calves. Give your hands a good shake.

2   Sitting in a circle, rub your hands together, then rub each shoulder using circular movements, rub your arms, your tummy, your thighs and knees.

3   Gently massage your cheeks using little circles, then your temples, then smooth away any frowns.

4   Put your thumbs at the back of your head and gently massage the top of your scalp with your fingers.

5   Standing or sitting, march up and down on the spot, really exercising your toes as you move. Then swing your arms back and forth as you march.

6   Circle your shoulder blades, first right, then left and then both together. First make a backward movement and then a forward movement.

7   Slowly turn your head from side to side, then shake your head a little more vigorously. Then move your head slowly and then a little faster.

8 Wrap one hand over the other and do a gentle stretch forwards, upwards. Then separate your hands, stretch and bring your hands down to your sides. (Please do not 'lace' your fingers as this can cause joint damage.)

9 Twist gently from the waist from side to side without forcing the movement. Allow your arms to swing by your sides.

10 Cup your hands and gently 'beat' up your arms and over your shoulders, tummy, and legs to stimulate your circulation.

11 Let your body go as floppy as possible (without falling over!) to really loosen those muscles.

12 Clench your fists and stretch your fingers alternately several times, then with both hands at the same time.

13 Wave to someone in the distance with one arm and then the other, and then with both arms together.

14 Shrug your shoulders gently at first, then see if you can touch your ears with your shoulders.

15 Try to rub your tummy with one hand and pat your head with the other hand. If you can, try it at a different pace (maybe tummy slow and head fast, for example).

Warm-ups with Names

16 Stand or sit in a circle, and take it in turns to say your names – then see if everyone can remember all the names! It usually takes a lot of practice.

17 Take it in turns to say the first letter of your name and see if the others can guess it; you can give clues such as 'it is also a flower' or 'a footballer has the same name'.

18 Using a soft ball, take it in turns to throw the ball and say your name. Then throw the ball and say the name of the person you are throwing it to. Finally throw the ball in the air and whoever catches it has to shout their name (for energetic groups only!).

19 Take it in turns to say your name and make a movement or gesture to go with it – then the rest of the group copies you like an echo. The movements don't need to be complicated.

20 Say your name and a food you like that starts with the same letter: 'My name is Mary and I love melon'.

21 Beat your chest vigorously and shout your name.

22 If your group has more than six people, then divide yourselves into smaller groups such as two groups of four, for example. In your group try to learn each other's names and say them in a rhythm like a chant, for example 'Sally, Jennifer, Freddie and Bill'.

23 Repeat the name chant and clap your hands at the same time.

24 Repeat the name chant and add a group movement that you all do together.

25 Place your hands on each other's shoulders and move in a circle to the name chant.

26 Say the name chant very quietly and slowly let it get louder and louder and then quieter and quieter until it becomes a whisper.

27 Repeat the loud and soft chanting but use the movement as well, so that the energy increases more and more and then decreases as the chant gets quieter.

28 Repeat the name chant and this time let it get faster and faster and then slow it down until it is like a slow motion drawl!

29 Repeat the name chant with a movement getting faster and faster, then slower and slower.

30 Share a name that you like instead of the one you have and play a name game with the new name.

Warm-ups with Breathing

Remember that developing breath control can help with panic attacks and asthma as well as being good for general well-being. When people practise breathing exercises they can feel a little giddy, so attempt the exercises at a gentle pace and stop if anyone gets too 'spaced out'.

Invite the group to do the following activities:

31 Breathe in through the nose and blow out through the mouth, pausing between each action.

32 Hold the right hand nostril closed by placing two fingers at the side of the nose – breathe in through the left nostril. Then hold the left nostril closed and breathe out through the right nostril. Repeat five times and then start the opposite way round with the left nostril.

33 Breathe in and out very noisily and notice how it sounds like the background noise to a film!

34 Be aware of your own breathing rhythm as you breathe in and out: do you 'panic' breathe in very fast gasps? Do you hyperventilate right down to the pit of your stomach? By breathing to a gentle in-out rhythm you can reduce anxiety.

35 Breathe in through the nose, wait for a count of four and blow out through the mouth, taking care not to let your breath out in a rush.

36 Be aware of the 'tummy up and bottom down' stance as this will help you to breathe easily and normally. Try the above exercises again and notice the difference when you stand (or sit) differently.

37 Breathe in with a series of four sniffs, hold for a count of four and then blow out through the mouth to a count of four. This exercise helps to develop your lung capacity.

38 The above exercise can slowly be increased but not too quickly or you will have very sore muscles between your ribs (the intercostal muscles). Increase by one sniff a week up to a count of eight. Any more and you will have the breathing capacity of an opera singer in the making!

39 This exercise is to help you sleep more easily and can be practised as a relaxation technique. Close your eyes as you sit back to back with a partner, or sit in a chair, or lie on the floor.

As you breathe gently in and out, picture the rise and fall of your own chest in your mind. You will notice that your breathing gets deeper and deeper and usually you will fall asleep.

40 Place your fingertips gently on your rib cage, take a deep breath and see if you can push your fingers away. If you can, it means you are expanding your chest outwards and not raising your shoulders. Raising your shoulders causes tension in your neck and only allows small intakes of breath.

41 Repeat this exercise, but this time place your hand on your diaphragm (just below your rib cage). Again, your hand should be pushed away as you breathe in.

42 If you repeat the exercise again and place your hand on your tummy, then it should not move away at all (you are keeping it flat – 'tummy up – bottom down', remember?).

43 To breathe in is also 'to inspire', so do not forget that you will have inspiration with correct breathing. Do any of these exercises again and remember to inspire!

44 Remember that you can use your breathing to indicate a mood – the disdainful sniff, the sharp intake of breath when scared, or the bored yawn – try them all out and think of some more.

45 Finally, the favourite! Imagine you are blowing up a balloon – hold it between your fingers and blow with deep breaths until it is as big as it will go. Tie the top, take an imaginary pin, count to three and burst it, shouting a very loud BANG!

Warm-ups with Voice

Some of the exercises in the Names section (such as nos 21 and 26) can be used for voice warm-ups. Humming exercises give confidence to people who are scared of opening their mouths. Voice warm-ups are really important to assist people to feel more confident and literally to 'find their voice'.

46 Hum until your lips start to tingle. Then hum again, stopping and starting.

47 Agree on a tune that everyone in your group knows and then hum it together.

48 As you hum, place your hands on your forehead and see if you can sense the vibrations of the hum, then on your cheeks, then on your neck and finally on your chest. Where do you feel the greatest vibrations?

49 Slowly hum up and down the scale (or la la) and be aware of when there is a change from a 'chest voice' to a 'head voice'.

50 Make a buzzing sound, very quietly at first and then louder. Imagine that a swarm of bees is in the distance and getting closer and closer!

51 Sigh loudly enough for everyone to hear (it helps with deep breathing). Allow it to develop so that you use your shoulders and arms as well.

52 Similarly, give a very noisy yawn with a stretch first upwards and then outwards.

53 Take some deep breaths and say la la la very quickly – it really gets the tongue moving!

54 Make the sound l, l, l, l, l, l, (six times) and say, la, at the end. Once this idea is established try it with other consonant sounds such as: m, m, m, m, m, m, ma; t, t, t, t, t, t, ta; p, p, p, p, p, p, pa; you can think up many more.

55 Practise very elongated vowels sounds: aaah – oooh – eeeh – aaay and so on. Then have a 'yodel' conversation with someone else in your group, just using vowels and gestures.

56 Have fun with tongue twisters: 'red leather, yellow leather'; repeat it slowly and then get faster and faster; or 'blue lorry, green lorry'; or 'thirty thrushes flew from Thetford to Russia'; or 'a laurel crowned clown'.

57 Recall a nursery rhyme and all sing it together; include rhymes from other cultures and countries. Teach it to those who do not know it.

58 Hum along to the music.
(A CD of rhythmic folk song melodies or popular songs that are easy to hum to is required for this activity.)

59 Sing along to the music. Take it in turns to sing a verse, either individually or in a small group.
(The words are needed for people who feel confident to sing words and maybe a chorus. There are simple folk songs from many cultures and indeed the melody can be the same with a change of words.)

60 Think of an entertainer and take it in turns to mimic their voice – either their speaking voice or their singing voice.

Warm-ups with Games

There is also a whole section on Play and Games (see p73). Here we have some simple warm-up games that can be used to energise the group and individuals, and make them ready for more developed work. Some games are for the whole group to do together, others are designed for pairs to interact.

61 (For the whole group.)
Touch a door handle, a window frame, two opposite corners of the room and shake hands with four people, all within two minutes. Then retrace your steps and see if you can remember who you shook hands with.

62 Take three giant footsteps, two hops, one jump and skip in a circle with a partner. Repeat three times – all within three minutes.

63 Walk briskly round the room without looking at anyone – in and out and not in straight lines.

64 Walk briskly round the room and make eye contact with everyone you meet.

65 Walk briskly round the room. Greet everyone using a made-up word as if it really exists (ie, believe in it).

66 Take your time to walk round the room and do a 'high five' with those people you encounter.

67 Get into a group with anyone who is wearing the same or a similar colour to you.
(There may have to be a group of mixed colours.)

68 When I call out two colours, touch one colour on yourself and one on somebody else.

69 (Again the theme of balloons (see no. 45, p40.) Make sure strong balloons are used. Cooperate as a group to keep the balloon in the air.
Then try to keep two balloons in the air at the same time.

70 Work in pairs and see if you can break the balloon by jumping on it.

71 Stuff a balloon up your jumper, then give your partner a hug and try to break the balloon.
(Use a lighter type of balloon – the clothing gives protection. For this technique women work with women and men with men.)

72 Draw a face on your balloon and say 'hello' to other faces.

73 Call out two body parts that it is OK to touch – for example 'chin to elbow' or 'toe to knee' – everyone has to join up with someone else.

74 Stand back to back with a partner and pretend to have an itch on your shoulders that you are going to rub against your partner's back.

75 With a partner, go for a walk while balancing on their feet – this involves some close hugs! If you feel confident doing this exercise, can you dance with your partner while standing on their feet?

Warm-ups with Games (2)

These games (nos. 76–9) are a little more complex and may involve more touching – only you can judge if your group is ready for them!

76 Hold a large balloon between two fingers and see if you can pass it to your partner without it floating away.

77 Hold an orange under your chin and see if you can pass it to your partner without dropping it.

78 With a partner, place your toes together, hold hands, straighten your arms and slowly lean back so that you are balancing each other.

79 Following the previous exercise with two people holding hands and balancing, add two people at a time, hold the waist of the person in front of you and lean back, so that eventually the whole group will be balanced. It is important to do this exercise slowly so that you lean back and balance each other at the same time.

80 Stand in a circle and all turn to your right, so you are standing one behind the other; on a signal, sit in the lap of the person behind you so that the whole group is doing a balanced sit.

81 (As people grow more confident in trusting another person, try number 78 again with this variation.) Once you are balanced, take one hand away – make sure you agree which hand! – then change hands, move from side to side, and sway up and sway down.

82 Stand in the circle and count 1, 2, 3 – on 4 everyone has to look at someone. If two people are looking at each other they change places. (It is a fairly fast moving game and the group leader needs to be watchful for the person who never gets looked at by anyone else.)

83 (If the group becomes confident with this game, introduce the idea of hats – there must be enough for everyone to have one and a few left over.)
Count to four again, but this time exchange hats as well as places when you meet someone's eyes.

84 Choose a hat and walk round the room in character of the person who would wear that hat.

85 Get into pairs and interact with each other. It will be more fun if you have two very different hats such as a flat cap and huge 'Ascot' hat.

86 Do the same, but add another item such as a shawl, a big bow, a bag or satchel and so on – something that you wear.

87 (A game inspired by Boal (1992) that has many names – 'hypnosis' will suffice.)
In pairs, one person holds their arm out, with the palm tilted up – their task is to move backwards round the room in various directions – the other person, as if hypnotised, follows the palm.

88 You have an imaginary wand and call out what your partner will turn into, BUT they turn into something else! Then interact.

89 Move about as if you are a dog or a wolf or a fox. Then make a group with animals that are like yourself – and see if you are right! Vary it with other animals or objects of a similar shape.

90 Let's all do the 'hokey-cokey' – really enjoy it and give it lots of energy.

Warm-ups with Feelings

Of course, all the other warm-ups will involve our feelings to a greater or lesser extent. However, the following techniques help people to clarify the expression of their feelings in appropriate situations.

91 'I am angry because ...' Complete the sentence and say it to a partner. For example, 'I am angry because I've lost my purse'. Your partner simply responds, 'You are angry'. Then it is your partner's turn.

92 (The group leader gives other examples of what makes them angry and the group discuss if the same things make them angry).
Now complete the sentence, 'I am not angry because ...' and your partner will say 'You are not angry'.

93 In small groups talk about something you find scary. Then 'own' the feeling, saying, 'I am scared of ...' or 'I feel frightened when ...'.

94 Choose something that has made you sad in the past and share it with the rest of the group. See if other people have had similar feelings of sadness.

95 'I feel very happy when ...' Everyone share something with the group and see if they can remember everyone else's happy moments.

96 In a group of three, play a game in which one person is angry, another is scared and the third is trying to reconcile the difference. Who starts to side with whom? (Usually the reconciler and the scared person stand together against the angry person.)

97 Repeat the exercise but this time the third person is a mediator and does not take sides but stays neutral.

98 Pull a face that expresses a feeling and the rest of the group have to guess what the feeling is. Adjust your expression if they get it wrong.

99 Look at some facial expressions in photos cut out of magazines and newspapers and see if the group can guess what the people are feeling.

100 Take a short headline cut out of a newspaper and mime it for the rest of the group to guess.

101 Using a pack of 'feeling' cards (such as the Feeling Card pack produced by Actionwork, see Resources), play a game where you enact the picture on the card and see if the group can guess what you are feeling.

102 Using the cards, have a group discussion about feelings and which ones you find difficult to manage.

103 Use the cards to make a continuum of shades of feeling – for example there are several that are about angry feelings that range from irritated to furious. Share different things that make you a little angry or very angry.

104 What colours would you use for your different feelings? For Anger? Sadness? Joy? Fear? Maybe use crayons or paints to give colour to feelings whether extreme or mild.

105 Use several pieces of paper to represent different feelings –
go round the room and colour your own feeling – see what
different colours the group ends up with.

106 Look at postcards of paintings or people and discuss what
feelings are being shown.

Warm-ups with Roles

These are brief role plays for people to start feeling more confident
about exploring roles; some of the earlier exercises such as 84 and
85 can also be used to warm up for roles.

107 Everyone has a piece of paper with a line on it – 'I am your
landlord – where is my rent?' 'I am your mother – why haven't
you called me? 'I am the doctor – where are your X-rays?' and
so on – in turn say a line to the person standing on your right
going round the circle. They do not respond – they just listen.

108 In pairs choose a sentence that appeals to you and let it
develop into a brief interaction.

109 In pairs one person says 'You must' and the other says 'I can't'
– let it develop into an interaction – that is all you can say.

110 In pairs and without words, one person looks defiant and the
other has eyes downcast – try it and then see what this scene
is about.

111 As a whole group, watch a football match very enthusiastically
with the right gestures and sounds.

112 You are all watching a film or television programme that is really disappointing and not what you expected – react.

113 In threes – one person is bursting to say something – another is saying 'Sssh' – another wants to know what it is!

114 In pairs – a salesman or woman at the door is trying to persuade you to buy something that you do not want.

115 In pairs – a shop where the sales person is trying to stop you buying something as it is reserved for someone else.

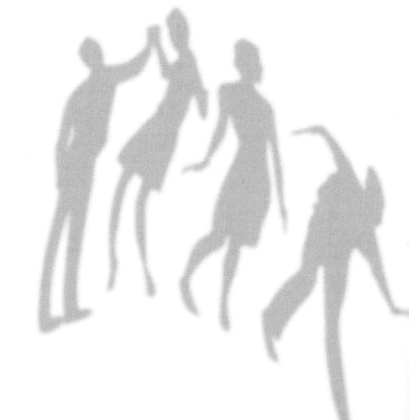

2 Movement and Relaxation

One of the most important things in your work is to be able to encourage people to MOVE; whether it is small steps or great big gestures, whether it is dancing in a circle or jumping for joy, movement is important. Adults as well as children need as many outlets for body-movement as possible and people will see that a lot of the warm-ups and games are very physical.

Some people have limitations because of physical illnesses, others are influenced by the medication they are taking, still more have a fear of movement because they are worried about their balance. The exercises in this section are a cross section for a variety of needs and abilities. You can always slow something down or make a simpler variation according to the needs of your particular groups.

Spend a few moments thinking about your own movement needs and whether you have physical tension or aching joints or generally feel ill at ease with your own body. Remember to move for yourself as well as for others!

A few cautions: make sure that people are in comfortable shoes for movement – slippers or high heeled shoes are equally inappropriate. Check that the floor is suitable for movement: wood or cork tiles are preferable to concrete. Make sure that individual people do not have a restriction on their movement because of a medical condition.

Having said that, remember that even the psalms encourage us to dance joyously and the Persian philosophers knew the importance of the dance, (see section 6, Stories and Documentaries, p139).

2.1 Relaxation and Deep Breathing

Group Size	small and medium
Materials	fleecy blankets, cushions or pillows
Duration	30 minutes

Encourage people to either sit on the floor on a cushion or to sit in a chair with a cushion behind their back. Give each person a fleecy blanket to tuck around themselves and allow them to find a position that is comfortable for them.

Suggest that they breathe in slowly through their noses and blow out the breath slowly through their mouths – let people find their own rhythm for this and slowly their bodies will relax more and more. They will often want to adjust their position once they feel more relaxed. Once you sense that the group is relaxed, slowly bring up some soothing music or sound effects from nature (there are several recordings of whale music that are popular).

Allow time for them to 'come back again' – five minutes before the end of the session suggest they slowly start to stretch, one limb at a time, starting with their fingers and toes until they can stretch their whole body. Then ask them to be aware of the light before they open their eyes. Finish the exercise by everyone removing their blanket and helping each other to fold it up.

Variations

- During the relaxing period, read people a story that is suitable for a calm atmosphere.

- Let people sit back to back if they can reach the floor, and relax supported by somebody else.

- Encourage people to share the most relaxing spaces and places they know.

2.2 Relaxing and Sleeping

Group Size	small and medium
Materials	fleecy blankets, cushions or pillows
Duration	30 minutes

Many people complain that they cannot sleep well. There are many reasons why people cannot finally 'drop off'. Maybe they are new to the hospital or home and it is all a bit strange, maybe they are used to being alert for partners and children. Some people find that worries about finances, or changes, or illnesses keep them awake until the small hours of the morning.

Encourage people to be comfortable on the floor or in the chair as in the last exercise. Then encourage the deep breathing exercise, breathing in through the nose and out through the mouth. Then suggest to people that they try and picture the rise and fall of their own chest as they are breathing deeply. Slowly people's breathing gets deeper and deeper and it is not unusual for them to fall asleep. As before, bring people slowly out of the relaxation and into an awareness of the room.

This is a safe exercise that they can do for themselves when they have difficulty falling asleep.

Variations

- Suggest to people once they are relaxed that they think of a safe place where they can sleep if they feel like it.

- Describe to people how they can imagine their comfy mattress, or maybe it is a real one that they still have, and that wonderful sensation as they climb into it and sink amongst the pillows and duvet.

- Invite people to bring along their favourite music for relaxing and share it with the group.

2.3 Swaying in the Wind

Group Size	any size
Materials	CD player, CDs of swaying music, for example, 'Blowin in the Wind'
Duration	10 – 15 minutes

Members of the group can sit or stand in a circle. They sway gently from side to side, keeping balance, hands by the sides. Suggest they hum the music and sway their arms from side to side.

Ask everyone to raise their arms and sway them from side to side over their heads.

Variations

- Give people light weight scarves to sway from side to side, making patterns.

- Suggest they hold the scarves in both hands and sway with their arms held high.

- Invite them to work with a partner and use two scarves to sway.

2.4 Fingers and Thumbs Keep Moving

Group Size	small and medium
Materials	none needed
Duration	10 minutes

Everyone sits in a circle; remind people of the tune of 'One finger one thumb keep moving'. Help people to learn the tune if they do not know it already.

Then learn the words: 'one finger one thumb keep moving', repeat three times and then add 'and so say all of us'. Slowly add on different body parts: 'one finger one thumb', 'one arm', 'one leg', 'one nod of the head'.

Then put the tune and the words and the actions together. It takes a little time to get going but it is a very valuable exercise for coordination and combining movement, voice and song.

Variations

- Invite group members to volunteer any action songs that they know and can teach the other members of the group.

- Sing a round such as 'Three blind mice' or 'London's burning' but do actions to the words.

- Repeat the same idea with words and actions to 'She'll be coming round the mountain ...'.

2.5   Circle Stretch

Group Size	small and medium
Materials	none needed
Duration	5 minutes

Bring everyone together in a circle and invite them to hold hands. They enlarge the circle as wide as possible and stretch their arms. Then they make the circle as small as possible. They stretch again but this time lift their hands high and lean back as far as they can. Do this exercise slowly so that everyone is balanced with everyone else. Repeat it once or twice so that people get used to coordinating together.

Variations

- Try this exercise with everyone sitting in a circle but follow the same sequence.

- Still sitting in the circle, everyone stretches up high and then bends forward low, still keeping hands held.

- Everyone holds hands, stretches high and sways from side to side.

2.6 Shake a Leg!

Group Size	small and medium
Materials	CD player and CDs
Duration	5 – 10 minutes

People can sit or stand in a circle. Choose some lively and rhythmic music and encourage people to clap along. They shake hands, one at a time and then both together. They shake one leg at a time from the knee downwards. They circle their ankles one at a time, and shake each foot alternately.

Everyone shakes as much of themselves as they can!

Variations

- Instead of shaking, encourage people to clap their hands and then slap their legs (good for circulation).

- Ask them to twist their waist from side to side and shake their shoulders.

- Sing along to 'Let's twist again like we did last summer'.

2.7 Dancing in the Circle

Group Size	small and medium
Materials	CD player and any CDs of traditional folk music
Duration	5 – 20 minutes

All folk music has a basic rhythm that allows for simple stepping. Invite the group to stand in a circle and hold hands. Suggest they step sideways to the right for two steps and then to the left for two steps. Establish this as the first sequence. Then try stepping forward for two steps and then back for two steps. These steps can be repeated in a slow sequence and then faster.

Variations

- Invite the group to repeat the sequence above but with a spring in their step.

- Start the dance with clapping first in order to establish the rhythm.

- Everyone faces the way they are going in the circle and instead of single steps, they do three running steps; they repeat this coming back the other way; three runs into the centre, then three runs coming out again.

2.8 Chain Gang

Group Size	small and medium
Materials	none needed
Duration	10 – 15 minutes

Invite people to stand in a circle and then ask them to pair off round the circle. Each pair face each other and shake hands with their right hand. They both move forward and shake hands with the next person with their left hands; they continue moving round the circle shaking alternate hands until they arrive back to their own partner.

Repeat the chain until people feel at ease with it.

Variations

- Use the folk music for people to move the chain round the circle.

- Suggest they skip as they move from right hand to left hand.

- Ask them to greet people as they shake hands with them so that they will have met half the group; they meet the other half by turning round and coming back the other way.

2.9 Moving with Hats

Group Size	small and medium
Materials	lots of different hats as varied as possible
Duration	20 – 30 minutes

You will find it useful to have a lot of different hats in your costume box: flat caps, baseball caps, straw hats, felt hats of all descriptions; additionally you can acquire jester's hats, veils and turbans. See the Drama and Role Play section (p117) for more uses for hats.

Initially you can invite people to choose a hat and if possible to look at themselves in a mirror. Suggest that they think about the person who might wear this hat and how they would move; walk round the room trying different walks and gestures; greet other people in the appropriate style. The emphasis is on the congruence between the movement and the hat and to encourage people to expand their movement.

Variations

- People put hats on their hands and use them as puppets instead of wearing them.

- Create a fashion show where everyone walks with very exaggerated movements.

- People dance with a partner in the style of the hat. (Formal? Traditional? Pop?)

2.10   Fun with a Parachute

Group Size	medium and large (depending on size of parachute)
Materials	medium play parachute with 12 or 18 handles
Duration	20 minutes

You will find a parachute a great asset and capable of bringing together very diverse groups. Adults are usually surprised how much they enjoy parachute play.

Everyone stands round the parachute and holds a handle; they slowly raise the parachute together and allow it to waft down. Slowly the group will get into a rhythm and be able to move the parachute together wafting up and down, and soon it will stay up longer as it fills with air.

Variations

- Play a game where people have to change places by running under the parachute: for example, everyone wearing red change places. There are always enough people to still hold up the parachute and the idea is to get to their new place before it comes down again.

- A tennis ball is put on top of the parachute and people roll it towards one another.

- Repeat the exercise with the tennis ball but this time it is rolled along specific colours such as 'red to green'.

2.11   More Fun with the Parachute

Group Size	medium and large
Materials	large parachute with 18 or 24 handles
Duration	20 minutes

This is a progression from the previous exercise and only undertaken when people feel comfortable with the parachute play. Always do the initial warm-up of wafting the parachute, then everyone sits down still holding the handles. Someone chooses to be a shark and two others choose to be minnows. The minnows move under the parachute and the shark is on top. Everyone else is shaking the parachute vigorously so it is difficult for the shark to find the minnows. Once 'caught' then new people become the shark and minnows.

Variations

- As above but this time there is a cat and mice: the mice are under the parachute and the cat is on top. People soon learn that if the mice are very still there is less chance of them being caught.

- The group stands up with the parachute and tries to keep an inflated beach ball in the air by moving the parachute.

- They allow the parachute to fill with air as they raise it up. Everyone sits down together in the middle of the circle and the parachute falls on them like a shelter.

2.12   Stretching the Borders

Group Size	small and medium
Materials	a strong circle of elastic rope
Duration	15 – 20 minutes

Suggest to group members that they all hold the rope and try
to pull it as hard as they can to expand the circle (it is important
to set ground rules that no one just lets go and causes others to
stumble). Now they stand inside the circle and press back to try
and stretch it again.

Variations

- Allow one person inside the circle to run and 'bounce' off the
  rope – they are supported by all the other group members
  holding the rope.

- Allow two people to do the same. They need to coordinate very
  carefully to make sure that they do not bump into each other.

- Alternately round the circle have one person inside and one
  person outside; the people on the outside hold the rope,
  the people on the inside relax against the rope.

2.13   Creating Small Group Movements

Group Size	small and medium
Materials	none required
Duration	20 minutes

Invite everyone to make small groups of three or four people.
First they share their names and then see if they can turn them into
a rhythmic chant. Then they decide on movements to fit this rhythm.
Each group puts the chant and movements together and shows it to
the other groups. They can then teach each other their chant dance so
that everyone can try all of them.

Variations

- Suggest to people that they vary the pace of the chant so that
  they can have slower movements as well as faster.

- As an alternative people can create a stamping dance to their
  name-rhythm.

- Put a sequence together for the whole group to do that
  incorporates everyone's names.

2.14   The New Machine

Group Size	small and medium
Materials	none required
Duration	15 minutes

Having done plenty of warm-ups to get the energy going, suggest to people that they are going to build a group machine. One person starts by standing in the centre and making a movement; another person comes and joins on and makes a synchronised movement. Slowly, one at a time, a whole machine is built up that is moving in a coordinated way.

Variations

- Suggest to people that they create a machine just using sounds.

- Put the sounds and the movements together to make a fully coordinated machine.

- Have someone as the person who starts up the machine by turning an imaginary switch: the machine starts very slowly and then gets faster.

2.15   Inventing a New Machine

Group Size	small and medium
Materials	none needed
Duration	10 – 15 minutes

Invite people to work in groups of three. They can move together as a machine using different body parts to be machine parts. They need to coordinate together so that the machine can really 'work'.

Variations

- Suggest to people that they are inventors and the machine does something quite specific.

- They create a machine that can go into outer space.

- They make a machine that can do boring jobs in a new and surprising way.

2.16   Moving with the Elements

Group Size	medium
Materials	pieces of large cloth in different colours
Duration	15 – 20 minutes

Choose one element at a time – Fire, Earth, Water and Air – and encourage people to move as the chosen element. First move with very small movements, then getting bigger and bigger before going small again. Then try the movements using the cloths: probably red for fire, green or brown for earth, blue for water and pale blue or white for air.

Variations

- Invite people to work with a partner using the material to create the elemental movement.

- In a small group they create two of the elements and let them interact.

- Let all the small groups interact and dance the elements.

2.17 Moving like Statues

Group Size	small and medium
Materials	large pieces of different cloth in different colours, coloured scarves
Duration	15 – 20 minutes

Invite people to work in pairs and one person swathes the other person in pieces of cloth to create a statue – but it is a statue that can move! The 'sculptor' then moves with the person and mirrors their postures. People then change over.

Variations

- Follow the exercise as described above but all the statues move together and interact with all the 'sculptors'.

- Link up all the statues with pieces of cloth so that they become one creation. People stay on the spot and move the rest of their bodies.

- Half the group create one sculpture with the other half of the group and then give it a title. Change over and repeat the exercise.

2.18　Dancing with Materials

Group Size	small and medium
Materials	different sizes of cloth but in light-weight fabric such as chiffon, CD player and CDs or a drum for rhythms
Duration	15 minutes

Invite people to choose a piece of cloth that is a colour they like. Suggest that they first of all play with the material – throwing it up in the air, waving it and so on. Then they move with their piece of cloth either to a slow gentle drum beat that changes in rhythm or to music sounds (for example, a CD of Reiki music is appropriate).

Variations

- Encourage people to move together once they have established their shapes and patterns.

- Vary the rhythm or music so that people dance or move to a faster beat, still using their materials.

- Suggest that people work in pairs or small groups and vary their movements between the faster and slower.

2.19 Moving Statues

Group Size	any size
Materials	drum or CD player and music
Duration	15 minutes

Using music or drum rhythm ask people to move round the room, in and out of everyone else, and when you give a loud drum beat (or stop the music) they stop and 'freeze' in a statue. You can suggest different ideas such as 'freeze like an animal' or 'freeze as a cat' or 'freeze as a child' (or elderly person). Then you unfreeze them and they continue moving until you stop them again.

Variations

- Suggest different moods that people can freeze into: angry, joyous, worried, scared and so on.

- People can create the statues of different sorts of weather: sunny, stormy, dull or rainy.

- Invite people to freeze as different fairy tale characters: a giant, a fairy, Red Riding Hood, the wolf – the group can also suggest ideas.

2.20   The Dancing Queen

Group Size	any size
Materials	CD player and CD of Abba music
Duration	15 minutes

The music of Abba is great for movement and dance with all age groups. The Dancing Queen especially is sure to get everyone 'on the move' and just put it on and let everyone move and dance as they wish. If they want to sing along as well, that is even better!

Variations

- Suggest that people really do dance as 'queen or king of the dance'.

- Use a CD of 'River Dance' in a similar way to encourage people in free movement and dance.

- Choose music with a strong rhythmic beat and suggest to people that they use the materials to dance with a partner.

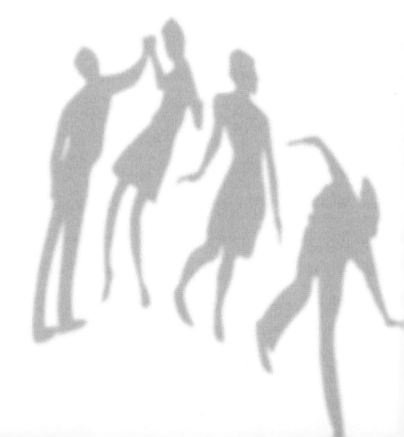

3 Play and Games

The two words 'play' and 'games' are often used interchangeably and this can cause so much confusion, especially as we say that we also 'play a game'. The easiest way to be clear about this is that games are created by human beings and they have a set of rules. The famous exception of course is when the game of Rugby was introduced when someone (William Webb-Ellis in 1823) *broke* a rule, running with the ball instead of kicking it, and the game of Rugby was born! Whereas play can be spontaneous or planned, personal or in groups, and often involves actions that mirror adult activities. So for example children will 'play at tea-parties' or 'play at monsters'; they will also play with things such as puzzles, art materials, dolls houses, sand and water. Something calculated to upset parents is when children 'play with their food'! If parents could view this as 'food as art' then perhaps it would be less stress making.

The following ideas include both play and games mainly for adults with a few ideas for teenagers and children included. The games are good for cooperation, setting limits and encouraging flexible and dextrous movement. However, there are people who have very bad memories of games at school and this type of activity can give rise to anxiety. Others will think that playing is childish and it is your job to encourage them to be playful and find their own creativity.

For many people their memories of games are competitive activities and they will be surprised that it is also possible to have cooperative games.

3.1 Newspaper Islands

Group Size	large
Materials	lots of old newspapers and CD player with music that can stop/start
Duration	10 – 15 minutes

Invite people to divide into small groups (two, three or four people); place a large sheet of newspaper for each group onto the floor and ask them to find a way for them all to be on the paper without touching the floor. This will involve some careful balancing and appropriate touch, and usually people start to laugh and 'fall off' their newspapers. It is a good 'ice-breaker'.

Variations

- Use hoops instead of newspapers.

- Use the hoops for a version of musical chairs and slowly take away one hoop at a time.

- As above but make the newspaper smaller!

3.2   Body Parts (1)

Group Size	large
Materials	none
Duration	10 – 15 minutes

Invite people to form small groups (three, four or five people).
Start the game simply by saying they can balance with only three
legs touching the floor (if it is a group of three). This is relatively
simple as people can just balance each other and stand on one leg.
The idea is to make it progressively more difficult and suggest for
example: two legs, four hands and a shoulder. This enables people
to really puzzle it out and solve the task. You can vary the body
parts depending on the mobility of the group.

Variations

- Use the same exercise but combine it with the previous one of
  Newspaper Islands.

- Invite people to create a moving statue with feet and arms
  joined together.

- Suggest that they move the statue but with balloons between
  their knees.

3.3 Body Parts (2)

Group Size	large
Materials	none
Duration	10 – 15 minutes

Divide the group into smaller units of five or six people.
The instructions need to be repeated more than once as initially people may think it is complicated. Explain that visible body parts have a number value, so that: backs count as 1, hands count as 5, bottoms 2, feet are 1 each. You can vary the number yourself if you wish. However, people usually remember hands as 5 because of 'high five'.

What is the largest score that each group can have touching the floor? It will take time for people to work this out and to find ways of helping each other to balance.

Variations

- Give the groups a specific numerical value to achieve, for example have only a maximum of six points touching the floor (two feet, two backs and one bottom).

- Reduce the number of points and see how ingenious people become.

- Vary the numbers in the group: you may find that you need to start with a smaller number, say three, while people get to know each other.

3.4 Word Pairs

Group Size	medium and large
Materials	cards
Duration	15 – 20 minutes

Prepare pairs of cards showing items that go together such as 'fish and chips', 'strawberries and cream', 'beer and skittles' so that you have a pack of pairs large enough for everyone in the group to have one card each. Make sure that members of the group are able to read.

Shuffle and then deal all the cards for people to have one each. They have to find their partner by shouting out the word on their card.

Variations

- Use the same game to work with opposite pairings such as 'hot and cold', 'night and day', 'tall and short'.

- Suggest to the group to move like their words rather than expressing them verbally. This is great fun and often leads to strange pairing.

- Encourage the group to create their own pairs on pieces of card and then use them.

3.5 Picture Pairs

Group Size	medium and large
Materials	cards
Duration	15 – 20 minutes

Create pair cards as in the previous exercise but instead of words use pictures of things that go together. This is helpful for people who have difficulty reading but also gives them some idea of the shapes of objects when they come to move the picture physically.

Lay all the cards out and invite people to look at all of them and then choose one for themselves. Then ask them to call out what the picture is and see if they can find their partner. Sometimes there is confusion when people think that a dog is a wolf or a cloud is a wig but fun ensues and it gives people a chance to be creative.

Variations

- People move round the room like their picture and find a partner who links with them in colour.

- Invite people to create small groups of pictures that have some links (maybe they are all animals, for example).

- Everyone mimes what is on their card to another person and if that person guesses correctly they can change cards and mime to another person until everyone has tried several cards.

3.6 Three Things (1)

Group Size	medium and large
Materials	none
Duration	15 minutes

This exercise is a move-on from the paired work that features in many of the exercises. Invite people to make groups of three. (If the group size does not divide into three then suggest groups of three or four.)

Ask them to find out three things that they have in common: it may be eye colour, favourite food, music, age and so on. The groups can then compare with each other if they shared similar things.

Variations

- Ask people to find things in common that are more specific such as hobbies, books, television programmes.

- People can also explore the complete opposite of their tastes such as music, films and so on.

- The small groups can mime what they share in common for the other groups to guess.

3.7   Three Things (2)

Group Size	medium and large
Materials	none
Duration	15 minutes

Invite people to form small groups of three or four persons. The task is to discover connections. What groups of three words go together, for example, 'Lock, stock and barrel'. Some people will think of sayings, others will think of objects such as 'knife, fork and spoon'. Either example is fine and they can then be shared in the bigger group.

Variations

- Discuss where these sayings come from such as 'Bell, book and candle'.

- Find three things that do not go together and see how it feels to say them.

- Discuss how many foods are grouped together because they 'belong'.

3.8 Fox and Lambs

Group Size	medium and large
Materials	hoops, newspapers and cushion or soft ball
Duration	15 – 20 minutes

Explain the game carefully and maybe a practice run is needed. One person is the fox and the remainder are lambs; the fox chases the lambs and tries to place a cushion (or soft ball) on one of their chests. Lambs can avoid this by running away or by hugging a partner but may only do that for a count of three. If you have the cushion or ball then you become the fox. Cushions may not be thrown!

Variations

- People can avoid being caught by standing inside the hoop or on the newspaper but only for a count of three.

- When the fox catches someone then they join hands until everyone in the room is a fox.

- People can escape turning into a fox by remembering the lambs' motto and saying it three times very quickly (the group decides what the lambs' motto is).

3.9   Stuck in the Mud

Group Size	medium and large
Materials	no resources needed (unless you try the variations below)
Duration	15 – 20 minutes

Everyone scatters round the room and one person is chosen to be 'it'. If someone is caught then they are 'stuck in the mud' and can only be released by someone else crawling through their legs. The aim of the person who is 'it' is to move fast enough so that everyone is stuck in the mud and no one can be rescued.

You may decide to have two people being 'it' if there are large numbers in the group.

Variations

- Once someone is 'stuck' then others have to stick on to them once caught and no one is freed.

- A person can only be 'stuck' if they are outside the hoops or the cushions.

- For people who are unable to run and chase they can be 'stuck' if they accept a rolled up newspaper (so they have to have arms and/or legs outstretched).

3.10 Tree Tig

Group Size	medium and large
Materials	none
Duration	10 – 15 minutes

Half the group become 'trees' and place themselves round the room. The other half scatter and are chased by the woodcutter. If the woodcutter catches someone then they freeze as an animal of the forest. They can escape being caught by sheltering with a tree – standing off the ground on their feet and holding on! But only for a count of three.

Variations

- Trees work in pairs and create a shelter round the escaping animal.

- The woodcutter tries to cut down trees (half the group) and has to stop if two people create a circle around him or her.

- Trees create a circle around the animal and the woodcutter tries to get inside the circle.

3.11 Grandmother's Footsteps

Group Size	medium and large
Materials	no equipment needed
Duration	10 – 15 minutes

This game is very good for encouraging concentration and physical control.

One person chooses to be grandmother and faces the wall at the end of the room. The other members of the group get to the opposite end and start to creep forwards, intending to be able to touch grandmother on the back without being seen to move.

Grandmother turns round every few seconds and points to anyone she can see moving and they have to go back to the beginning. As grandmother turns round everyone should 'freeze' to avoid being sent back.

The first person to go the length of the room without being seen to move now becomes grandmother.

Variations

- Two people move together towards grandmother.

- Energetic people might try the game on their hands and feet!

- People are only allowed to take huge steps.

3.12 What's the Time Mr Wolf?

Group Size	medium and large
Materials	none
Duration	10 minutes

One person chooses to be Mr Wolf and faces the wall at one end of the room and the remainder of the group creep up behind him. As they advance they call out 'What's the time, Mr Wolf?' In reply, Mr Wolf calls out a time. When he calls out '12 o'clock and time to eat you up' he or she chases the others and if anyone is caught they then become Mr Wolf. As in the previous exercise it is a game that requires control and concentration.

Variations

- Try the same game but dividing the group in half – one half are the Mr Wolves and the other half creep up. The wolves need to cooperate regarding the time!

- Some of the group hold hands, stand in a line across the middle of the room and alternately raise and lower their arms as the wolves try to capture the rest of the group.

- Change Mr Wolf into Mr Tiger (as they play in Malaysia) and add the snarls of the tiger.

3.13 Remembering What's in the Basket

Group Size	small and medium
Materials	none
Duration	10 – 15 minutes

Everyone sits in a circle and you explain the game carefully as some people may not have played it before. Suggest the idea of holidays and what people might bring back from a holiday. In the imaginary basket (or you might choose to have a basket as a prop) everyone decides what they brought from holiday. The game starts with the first person, 'I went on holiday to Greece and brought back some olives ...' The next person says 'I went to Spain and brought back some castanets, and some olives from Greece ...'

Each person chooses a country and has to also remember all the other things that people have said. The last person in the circle has a lot to remember.

Variations

- Focus just on food from different countries (or from different counties in the UK).

- Choose one country and bring back something that starts with the same letter: Denmark – I brought a dog, a diamond, and so on.

- Change it to a seasonal topic such as Christmas or birthdays, and say the gifts received that are in the basket.

3.14   Guessing Feelings

Group Size	small and medium
Materials	pieces of paper with different feelings and moods written down: angry, sad, clown-like, furious, confused
Duration	15 – 20 minutes

The group choose a phrase such as 'Many hands make light work'. They take it in turns to pick up a piece of paper and say the phrase in the feeling or mood that is written on the paper. The rest of the group have to guess what mood or feeling is being expressed.

Variations

- Each person walks like someone experiencing that feeling or mood (often less scary for people unused to creative work) and the rest of the group guess.

- Instead of saying a phrase, the person has to mime the feeling that is on the paper and the group guess what feeling it is.

- Have two or three groups; one representative from each group comes to you to get the piece of paper – they say the phrase and if the rest of their group get it right, they can go and fetch another feeling. The first group to finish all the feelings is the winner.

3.15 Change the Baton

Group Size	small and medium
Materials	a stick (without splinters!)
Duration	20 minutes depending on the size of the group

It is important that a gentle pace is established for this exercise as people need 'thinking time'. You explain to the group that the baton can become whatever they would like it to be and you can demonstrate one example such as playing it like a flute. Then pass it round the group and everyone thinks of something and the others guess what they are doing. You need to be careful that it does not turn into a situation where people feel they have to be very 'clever' with their ideas.

Variations

- If passing the baton round feels too confrontational, then leave the stick in the middle and people can pick it up when they have thought of something.

- Invite people to create something very big with it and conversely something very small, for example using the baton to paint their fingernails.

- Suggest group members use it as something that involves another person such as a fishing rod that catches a fish (the other person).

3.16 Change the Object

Group Size	small and medium
Materials	cushion or plastic bowl
Duration	20 minutes

Place the object in the middle of the circle and encourage people to use it as something that is new. So a cushion could become a TV set, a shower head, a loaf of bread, for example. Other members of the group have to guess what it is. As in the previous exercise it is important that it stays simple and that people do not compete to choose something too clever.

Variations

- Invite people to divide into pairs and work on an idea together and then show it to the group.

- Suggest that the cushion could be something that is alive.

- Invite the group to choose only something that is mechanical.

3.17   Mime the Object

Group Size	small and medium
Materials	none
Duration	20 minutes

People can stand or sit in a circle for this game and a lot will depend on the mobility and age of the group. One person mimes an imaginary object and then passes it to the next person. They turn it into something else and pass it on again. The object changes each time it is passed on to another person. See how many different items are mimed by the end of the group. The 'object' is not passed on until the group have guessed what it is.

Variations

- When the person receives the object they have to use it in the same way before changing it.

- They can keep the object the same all the way round the circle but use it in a different way when they receive it.

- They can try using the object as something completely different from what it is supposed to be for.

3.18   Houdini Escapes Again

Group Size	small and medium
Materials	none
Duration	20 – 30 minutes

Invite people to be in small groups of four or five. Each group decides on a situation from which it would be very difficult to escape. They give the scenario (written down or tell it) to another group who have to plan their escape. The ground rule is that they have to choose appropriate things: for example they could not have a bulldozer in the middle of the jungle where they are trapped. Each group actually tries out their escape plan and then shares it with the others.

Variations

- People plan the escape but are only allowed three objects to help them.

- They create an escape from another planet so special objects are allowed.

- Instead of escape FROM somewhere, people think of escaping TO somewhere.

3.19 Games with Cards

Group Size	small and medium
Materials	packs of cards of different types (see Resources)
Duration	30 – 40 minutes

It is really important that we do not underestimate the value of different card games. Most people will be familiar with conventional card games from Snap to Whist and a few others in between. Since people are already familiar with card games it is easier to introduce other card games. There is a wide variety of cards that address our feelings (in particular Actionwork) and they can be used to talk about feelings. For example, group members draw a card from a pack and share within the group whether they experience that feeling or whether they know others who may have a similar feeling.

Variations

- Invite group members to choose a card and mime the feeling and others have to guess what it is.

- They choose a card and say when somebody would express that feeling.

- They choose a card and say when it would be appropriate to express the feeling and when it would not!

3.20   Games on Boards

Group Size	small and medium
Materials	a variety of board games
Duration	20 – 30 minutes

As with the previous exercise, it is easy to forget the value of conventional board games and we need to remember that for many people they are familiar and create feelings of security. Unless of course you are the sort of person that never got the hang of a game and so felt a bit undermined. Some board games need skill and take more time and others are purely chance. They are very good for getting people to interact with each other and to feel they have something tangible to do. I am not suggesting that that is all we do but often it is a good starting point.

Variations

- Encourage people to share the games they played as children and things they liked and disliked.

- Create a game where the group have to solve a mystery through a series of clues that is less a board game but more a group exercise to solve.

- Create a story about a game competition such as 'Chess Championship' where something very unexpected happens.

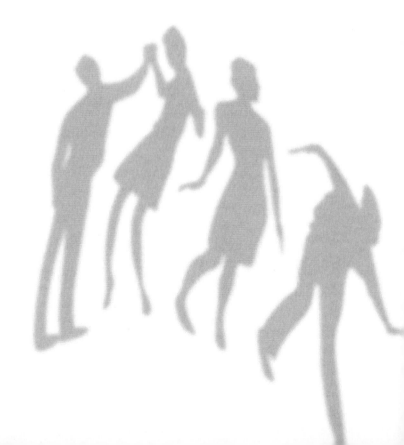

4 Pictures and Images

This section can be described in the broadest sense as 'using art', ie visual and tactile materials such as paint, finger paints, crayons, felt-tipped pens, pastels, paper and glue, clay and dough, Plasticine, newspapers and magazines, plaster bandage (Mod-Roc), glitter glue, felt and foam, card, dried leaves and flowers. Many people feel safer with tangible materials that they can sit and organise. These techniques assist people to expresss their feelings and ideas in different materials and to give form to them.

Many of these materials can be available at little or no cost, and the more we can recycle the more we are contributing to a more sustainable society. It is a challenge to always ask 'Can we use it?' before throwing stuff away. I always remind people of the National Theatre whose budget for props had run out; they needed a lavish set to depict the riches of the Incas for a play 'The Royal Hunt of the Sun' by Peter Shaffer. The Stage Manager sent his assistant on a visit to the local pubs to collect metal bottle tops – and these were subsequently beaten to make the most exquisite ornaments, plates, jugs and so on. Nobody guessed their origin and everyone gasped at the splendour of the set! You can also get inexpensive art materials from your local 'scrap store'; local firms donate leftover fabrics, metals and so on and the paints and brushes are very cheap.

Working with these materials is usually termed 'Projective Activities, (see Jennings, 2006 for a more detailed description) and developmentally the activities come after physical and embodied techniques (see Part 1, p2).

Some people need to be reassured that they do not have to be 'good at art' to enjoy artistic playing; other people feel more comfortable starting with something very tangible. Only you know what feels right for your group.

Any exercise marked with an asterisk (*) can be used either as a warm-up to more complex activities or in its own right.

4.1 Self-portrait (1)

Group Size	for individuals or small groups
Materials	paints, crayons or pencils, A3 size paper
Duration	30 minutes +

Invite people to close their eyes and think about how they see themselves in a positive light. Ask them to imagine that there is a commission to paint their portrait – what would you like to be wearing in the picture?

Ask everyone to open their eyes and to create a portrait of themselves. They can choose what they are wearing. When everyone has finished, they can share the pictures with each other and consider different people's perspectives.

Discussion
In which part of a gallery would I like my pictures to be hung?

Variations

- Group members decide on a background or landscape for their portrait.

- They imagine they live in a stately home and create a portrait that would be in the hall.

- They create their portrait as if they are a famous character from a book or film.

4.2 Self-portrait (2)

Group Size	for individuals or small groups
Materials	each person has an A4 piece of card, a portrait photo of themselves, felt-tipped pens and a round or oval stencil to cut out a hole in the middle of the card, scissors and masking tape
Duration	40 minutes

Invite people to carefully cut out an oval or circular hole in the middle of the card that is smaller than the photograph. They should draw a frame round the oval or circle using any pattern they like (for example wavy or squiggly lines; plain or double lines). Then they can decorate the four corners of the card in any way they like with colours of their own choosing. Finally, they stick their portrait using masking tape on the back of the card. They now have a decorated portrait of themselves.

People can share the portraits with each other and possibly create a portrait gallery.

Discussion
How important are photographs to us? Do we have many pictures from long ago?

Variations

- Do the same exercise but with pictures of group members when they were babies or children.

- Instead of decorating the card, people can write down on the card things that are important to them. For example, in one corner they could write down their favourite foods, in another their favourite books and films, colours, flowers and so on.

- Each group member writes their name in fancy handwriting underneath their portrait.

4.3 Self-portrait (3)

Group Size	for individuals or small groups
Materials	old newspapers, scissors, pencils, glue, A4 paper
Duration	45 minutes +

Invite people to draw a head and shoulders outline and then tear up pieces of old newspaper. Suggest they glue them within the outline to make a collage portrait of themselves. Encourage people to experiment with this rather than showing them one that is completed, otherwise they are likely to copy it! People might cut out features from the newspaper to create their face but the idea is to make the face from pieces – so several pieces for the hair – not just someone else's hair. People can get quite adventurous with this medium.

Share the new style portraits and methods used in the group.

Discussion
How did it feel to tear the paper and use it rather than cut it out more precisely?

Variations

- Use A3 paper and do a group collage portrait. When the group have finished, suggest they decide on a name for the portrait.

- Each group member cuts out actual words from the newspapers and makes a portrait with the words (group leader to check that people do not concentrate only on negative words). Have these words ever been used to describe them?

- Suggest they cut out several faces and use them to create a picture of themselves from different viewpoints.

4.4 Newspaper Poems

Group Size	any size
Materials	old newspapers, felt pens, scissors, pencils, glitter glue, A4 paper
Duration	30 minutes

Choose a theme, such as 'the weather' or 'grandmother' or 'memories'. Invite people to create a poem by cutting out words from the newspapers and sticking them on paper. The poem can be as long or short as they like. When they have written the poem they can then decorate it with colours or glitter glue.

When everyone has finished people can read their poems in the group and words of encouragement can help them write more poems.

Discussion
How words communicate the pictures in our mind.

Variations

- Suggest to people that they create a poem around any theme they choose.

- Groups of three people create a poem together on a given topic.

- Individuals create an angry poem about something they cannot tell anybody.

4.5 Playing with Paint (1)*

Group Size	small
Materials	different colours of paint, stubby paint brushes or small pieces of cloth tied over the end of sticks. Any size paper
Duration	15 – 20 minutes

Encourage people to play with the colours using stubby style brushes; they can make patterns and swirls, and it does not matter if the colours run into each other. Thinner paper will make holes very quickly so try to use card from packaging or boxes. The main aim is to free people to play rather than paint in formal styles. They will always joke about creating modern art and not being as good as their children can do. Just allow everyone to have fun including yourself!

All the pictures could then be placed together to create the idea of modern wallpaper.

Discussion
How does it feel to be so free with your paint? Breaking the rules?

Variations

- Introduce the idea of creating a patchwork quilt and everyone has a diamond shaped piece of card to play with; then place them all together.

- Use a large piece of paper for the whole group to sit round and make a group picture using the colours in the same way.

- Ask people to write their names in many colours using stubby brushes.

4.6 Playing with Paint (2)*

Group Size	any size
Materials	small sponges, several bowls with paint, card
Duration	35 minutes

Similar to the previous exercise, this is good for freeing people to just experiment rather than feeling they have to reproduce something specific. Sponges are great for making patterns and also squeezing to make trickles or blobs of paint. Sponges are easier to control than brushes so many people feel more comfortable with them. It does not work if the paint is too runny: try thickening it with cornflour or last year's suntan cream!

These sorts of exercises cause lots of mess so be ready with the wipes and cloths.

Variations

- Have large pieces of card, for example from big boxes, and use big sponges to make colours and patterns.

- Protect the floor and put a large piece of paper on the wall: the group can throw small paint sponges to make an action picture.

- Group members create a sponge picture using their opposite hand and see what happens.

4.7 Playing with Paint (3)*

Group Size	any size
Materials	large pieces of card, thick paint brushes, (at least 7.62cm), large tubs of paint
Duration	30 minutes

Invite people to paint in broad brush strokes rather than tiny details; you or they can suggest a theme. Broader brushes often give people more confidence to play with paint and they can build up several layers if they wish. Card is more absorbent and gives a firm surface at the same time.

Variations

- People can cover their card with paint and then use a wooden stylus or end of a paint brush to create a picture.

- Suggest they use the card to make any three-dimensional shape and paint in the same way.

- Use large boxes (such as TVs and refrigerators are packed in) to create a large construction for the whole group to paint – they may use even larger brushes.

4.8 Playing with Colours (1)*

Group Size	suitable for all group sizes
Materials	lots of different coloured felt-tipped pens and large paper or card
Duration	30 minutes

Invite people to choose pens of their two favourite colours and, holding both pens together, try to write their name with both colours at the same time. It will take a little practice and then their name looks really great! Once they are pleased with it, they can colour the background in shading and patterns.

Variations

• Create a group collage with everyone's name written in this style.

• Be daring and try writing with three pens!

• Each person writes their name with one colour and decorates it with leaves and flowers using other colours.

4.9 Playing with Colours (2)*

Group Size	individuals and medium groups
Materials	Finger paints or safe acrylic paints thickened with sand or hand cream, card or thick paper, scissors, wipes and kitchen roll
Duration	45 minutes (depending on 'engagement')

Invite the group to experiment using their fingers rather than paint brushes; it is very important that this is invitational as messiness makes some people feel very uncomfortable. Rather than having a fixed theme, suggest that people see what the paint does as they play with shapes, patterns and colours.

Discussion

Invite people to talk about the feelings of using their finger with the paint and how they achieved a picture.

Variations

- Suggest that everyone makes their thumbprint on a shared piece of paper – examine all the differences in people's 'marks'.

- Finger paint a tree of any sort and then cut it out; stick it on a large piece of card to create 'the forest of the group'; be sure to let people place their tree where *they* want it to be, not where you think it looks better!

- The group chooses a theme and everyone finger paints their own ideas.

4.10 My Hands, My Feet (1)

Group Size	small and medium
Materials	Vaseline, 'Mod-Roc', scissors, lots of newspapers, plastic bottles that spray water, wipes, clear varnish (optional)
Duration	50 minutes

People may need a demonstration of how this works before they start themselves. Cut a piece of the Mod-Roc larger than your hand; cover your hand with a thin layer of Vaseline; place the Mod-Roc on the back of your hand and spray water over it. When it is all wet you can mould it to the shape of your hand, smooth it and wait a few moments for it to dry. Gently peel it off your hand and wait for it to dry hard – if it is placed in the sun or you have a hairdryer that can take a few minutes. Otherwise you will need to let it dry until the next session. Clean the Vaseline and any plaster bits off your hand.

Group members decide how they want to paint their hand and use thick colours. The hands can be varnished if they wish.

Variations

- Invite people to follow the same procedure to make a model of one of their feet.

- They can model their hand and then create a landscape on the back of their hand as well.

- Suggest they create the hand of a 'model' with long tapering fingers or some other character they can think of.

4.11 My Hands, My Feet (2)

Group Size	small and medium
Materials	newspapers, card, paints or crayons, pencils
Duration	40 – 50 minutes

Invite people to draw round one of their hands and then ask them to look at the shape of it. Suggest that their hand could become something else and then invite them to turn it into something else by colouring or painting. For example, I have seen people turn their hand into a swan, a tree, a bunch of flowers. People often surprise themselves at the transformation of the basic shape and gain a lot of satisfaction from their own creative ideas.

Discussion
Discuss and share similarities between group members' pictures.

Variations

- Try the same exercise with a footprint.

- Suggest everyone turns their hand into a bird and create a bird collage.

- Use hand prints to create a large group tree.

4.12   Peas and Beans and Melon Seeds

Group Size	small and medium
Materials	old newspapers, card, PVI glue, glue brushes and a variety of seeds, lentils, split peas, melon seeds, beans, tweezers if possible
Duration	45 – 55 minutes

Invite each group member to think about a picture or pattern they can create with a mosaic of seeds and so on. They paint a thin layer of glue on the card and then group shapes of seeds to make the picture. Tweezers help to make it a little easier to place the seeds, but fingers, especially for beans, are fine. And remember how many different shapes and colours in beans there are: but the heavier the bean the more glue will be needed. If the glue dries before the picture is finished then paint on another layer, maybe a patch at a time.

Variations

- Do the same procedure but aim to create a group picture, the group having decided on the theme first.

- Invite them to draw a picture on the card, say of an animal or flower, and then glue it and place the seeds and beans.

- Group members write their name, glue it and decorate it with seeds and beans.

4.13   Magazine Collage: Diversity *

Group Size	any size
Materials	a variety of old magazines, catalogues and supplements, scissors, glue sticks, A4 paper or card
Duration	50 minutes

Invite people to cut out many different human figures and create a collage of a large crowd of different people: ages, gender, disabilities, races, costumes and so on. The idea is to create diversity.

Discussion

Invite people to comment on the balance of pictures they found in the magazines and how representative it is of our society.

Variations

- Suggest that people make a collage of lots of different shelters and houses.

- Create a group collage of holiday scenes.

- Create a collage of a street with different houses, gardens, people and pets.

4.14   Colour My Feelings (1)

Group Size	individuals or small groups
Materials	card or paper, crayons, pastels or coloured pencils
Duration	35 minutes

Invite people to choose different colours to represent their different feelings. Suggest they create a picture that includes all their feelings in it as a pattern with colours and shapes.

Discussion

Share differences in people's ideas for different colours.

Variations

- Encourage group members to create shapes for different feelings (circles, squares and so on) and colour them.

- Suggest they make the outline of a person and place the colours where the person experiences the feelings.

- Invite people to colour a landscape that has all the elements and link them with feelings; for example is the fire angry or happy?

4.15 Colour My Feelings (2)

Group Size	individuals or small groups
Materials	card or thick paper, crayons, pastels or felt-tipped pens, 22cm circle template
Duration	35 minutes

Provide everyone with two circles and invite them to create their happy face on one and their less happy face on the other, especially using colours to indicate how the faces are feeling. Look at the differences between the two faces and the use of colour.

Discussion

Invite people to share their faces and talk about when they feel happy and less happy; does anything trigger a change from one to the other?

Variations

- Suggest that people create a happy face and an angry face and look at what makes them change.

- Invite them to create a happy face and a miserable face and look at what makes them change.

- Using smaller circles, create a group collage with all different faces with feelings.

4.16 Clay or Dough – Making Anything (1)

Group Size	small
Materials	modelling clay or dough, card
Duration	35 minutes

Give everyone a piece of clay (preferably) or dough (have some spare flour ready in case it gets sticky) about the size of a small fist. Use the card as a clay-board. Invite people to close their eyes and to play with the clay: pat it, squeeze it, roll it and so on. Then make a shape, still with eyes closed. It does not have to be of anything in particular. When they open their eyes and look at what they have created, most people are usually very surprised. Once dry the creation can be painted if people wish.

Discussion

What was it like to work with your eyes closed?
Share anxieties about not being 'good enough' and take pleasure in your own creativity.

Variations

- Start in the same way and then invite everyone to make something from outer space.

- Start in the same way and invite everyone to make a model of a feeling.

- Work as a group with eyes open and create a model of a landscape.

4.17 Clay or Dough – Make Something (2)

Group Size	individuals and small groups
Materials	modelling clay or dough, spatula or small stick, card
Duration	35 – 40 minutes

Invite the group to press the clay flat on the card so that it makes a surface for working on. They can use the spatula or stick to create different shapes and patterns in the clay; they can always smooth it over and start again. They should end up with a pattern they like that uses many different types of indentation.

Variations

- Suggest that they draw the outline of a tree or animal and then use the spatula to create different textures as a way of 'colouring' in the image.

- People can use the spatula to create a landscape in the clay with different textures and shapes.

- Invite everyone to model the clay in 3-D to create a landscape and paint it when it has set.

4.18   Clay and Dough – Making Specifics (3)

Group Size	small
Materials	clay and card
Duration	35 – 45 minutes

All people to have a fist-size piece of clay and let the group choose a theme. Everyone creates their own model linked to the theme. Encourage people to respect and accept each other's models. Once they are really dry they can be painted with acrylic paints. Do the models all relate to each other as a collection?

Variations

• People can try the above exercise with their eyes closed.

• Group members make a model of a head and shoulders of anyone they choose.

• They can make use of the clay to model a name plate and then paint it when dry.

4.19   Paint a Poster

Group Size	small and medium
Materials	A3 size paper, paints, pencils and crayons
Duration	50 – 60 minutes

Invite everyone to think of a great time in their lives in the recent or distant past. Discuss how there are posters to promote special events, and ask what sort of posters catch their eye? What do they really notice? Then suggest they create a poster of the special event in their lives and create it in a style whereby it is eye-catching. Create an exhibition where all the posters are stuck on the wall and people look at everyone else's as well as their own.

Discussion

What does it feel like to have your life on the wall? Is there anything more about this special event you would like to share?

Variations

- Invite group members to make a small poster instead of a birthday card for a friend.

- Suggest they create a poster from pictures and words from magazines.

- They could try making a poster for something really silly instead of something important!

4.20   Make a Certificate

Group Size	medium size
Materials	card, scissors, coloured crayons, pencils and pens
Duration	30 – 60 minutes

Invite members of the group to close their eyes and focus on their achievements in the past: they may be small steps in a difficult life. For example, learning to walk again after an operation or cooking a meal for the first time. There are many things that people have achieved in their lives for which they have not been praised or rewarded. Suggest that everyone chooses something for which they will create a certificate. They can then make a certificate for themselves with the right wording and an appropriate picture or drawing, or even stick a red ribbon like a rosette.

Variations

- Each person shares memories of achievements for which they were rewarded.

- Each person creates the certificate they also hope to get!

- Each person creates a certificate for just being themselves, and a very special individual.

5 Drama and Role Play

Many people are nervous of role play and drama and think they might be made to feel stupid. Often it dates back to school days when we were made to stand up in front of a class and felt very exposed or ridiculed. There are stages of getting into roles and we need to work at it gradually with people. I suggest that you always attempt lots of warm-ups and movement before making that transition into role playing of any kind. The statue exercises in the Movement and Relaxation section (p51) are especially helpful.

Role play and drama can be used in several different ways. The most important question to address is whether you intend your group to practise life and social skills or whether you wish to encourage the development of their own creativity and imagination. I think that both are important so that the drama can be both a rehearsal for living as well as a means of expanding our own awareness and creativity.

All the exercises can be adapted (as with everything else in this book) to suit different age groups and different mobility capacity. Never feel that anyone is too old or too ill or too immobile to participate in creative work.

5.1 Focus on Faces

Group Size	small and medium
Materials	none required unless you do the mirror exercise
Duration	10 minutes

Invite people to massage their own faces and to feel all the different shapes of their cheeks, eyebrows and so on. Then ask people to frown, to frown upwards, to give a very big smile, to press their lips closed as if they refuse to speak and so on. Then name different expressions for people to show: an angry face, a miserable face, a confused or lost face. Take it slowly through different expressions and allow people time to 'change their face'.

Variations

- Invite people to make a sound when they make the face that also expresses the feeling.

- Suggest to members of the group that they can practise the face in the mirror and then show it to the group.

- Encourage people to create a face of their own choosing and the others have to guess what the expression is.

5.2 The Human Mirror

Group Size	small and medium
Materials	none required
Duration	10 – 15 minutes

Invite people to make pairs and to stand opposite their partners.
One person is the 'mirror' and the other person is looking in the
mirror. The mirror copies everything the other person does as they
are looking in: they may be pulling faces or putting on make-up or
looking at their tongue. Usually everyone at some point squeezes a
spot! Ask the people who are looking in the mirror not to move too
quickly or the mirror won't keep up!

Variations

- Suggest to the person looking in the mirror that they are opening
  a medicine bottle, taking a teaspoon, and drinking some very
  nasty medicine.

- Invite everyone to slowly put on a very special hat or necktie
  or other piece of clothing that shows they are going
  somewhere special.

- Encourage people to develop their own ideas of being a
  'character' when they look in the mirror: maybe a burglar
  or a chef or ...

5.3 Puppets on Strings

Group Size	small and medium
Materials	CD player and CD of 'Puppet on a String' or similar
Duration	15 minutes

Invite people to make pairs and make sure that everyone is physically warmed up. The pairs face each other; one person 'moves the strings' and the other moves like a marionette puppet. Explain to the group to keep it a simple puppet so move either a knee, or an elbow or a hand or the head. When people feel comfortable they can move their puppet round the room.
Then change round.

Variations

- Suggest to group members that they alternate hands and feet when moving their puppet to encourage it to dance.

- One person stands behind their partner on a rostrum or low platform; their partner moves their limbs and the person on the platform has to closely follow to look as if they are moving the strings.*

- Let the puppets meet each other and do a dance.

*This is especially positive for people with disabilities because they dictate the movement rather than the puppeteer.

5.4 A Play about Puppets

Group Size	small and medium
Materials	dressing up cloth pieces, hats, scarves
Duration	30 minutes

Bring the group together after a warm-up to have a discussion. Encourage people to think of the stories about puppets: Pinocchio, Coppelia ... Suggest that they make up their own puppet story (NB this is not a story that uses puppets, they are in the 'Puppets and Masks' section p155). Maybe it is someone who is turned into a puppet or the other way round. Maybe people could work on the story in small groups of four or five and then share their puppet drama with the whole group.

Variations

- Suggest that people dance as a puppet and their partner is their shadow and follows them.

- Invite people to make up a more personal story about someone who was manipulated as a puppet, and then create a drama.

- Encourage group members to find pictures (on the internet) of the traditional puppet dramas in India and China and use costumes or cloth to turn themselves into one of these huge puppets and move as one of the characters.

5.5 Drama and Sculpting (1)

Group Size	small and medium
Materials	none needed
Duration	15 minutes

Explain to people what we mean by a 'body sculpt'; ie a person or people are grouped according to a theme or a role or a scene. Sculpts can be 'free' – you just stand there how you choose – or someone creates a sculpt using other people, or a small group create a sculpt themselves. It is like a photograph of here and now feelings.

Suggest that everyone places themselves in the room to indicate how they are feeling. This is a free sculpt that can become a scene as you notice sub-groupings, isolation and people indicating different moods and attitudes through their body posture.

Variations

- Invite people in pairs to create a sculpt that shows two opposite feelings – for example, 'happy and sad'; or other opposites like 'small and tall'.

- Suggest that people work in groups of three or four and create a sculpt of a holiday scene.

- The same exercise but a holiday scene that went wrong!

5.6 Sculpting and Drama (2)

Group Size	small and medium
Materials	large cloths, hats and scarves
Duration	30 minutes

Encourage the group to choose a theme that could be the title of a play. If the group are new to these activities then keep it simple, for example 'Murder Mystery at the Tower'. Once people have decided on the broad outline of the story then suggest they make a sculpt of the beginning, middle and end in small groups and then share with the rest of the group.

Variations

- Repeat the above exercise but suggest they create the sculpt and wear the costumes.

- Repeat the exercise and now the characters in the sculpts each say one word.

- Finally invite people to let the sculpt lead into a short scene, and perhaps each small group is responsible for one scene in the play.

5.7 Sculpts and Metaphors

Group Size	medium and large
Materials	pieces of cloth and a book of quotations
Duration	30 minutes

Encourage people to think of a metaphor that describes the whole group or the institution or school. For example, someone might say 'this school is like a prison'. Suggest they create a sculpt to represent the prison metaphor and integrate everyone's perceptions. People always discover that they understand something better by sculpting it.

Variations

- Suggest people create a sculpt to illustrate what the group would look like if it was on another planet (Major Tom to Ground Control!).

- Invite the group to think of a metaphorical saying, such as 'All work no play makes Jack (or Jill) a dull boy', for example; create a whole group sculpt of the saying.

- Take a famous proverb or saying, or quotation such as Shakespeare's 'To be, or not to be – that is the question' and create a group sculpt.

5.8 Sculpts and Everyday Life

Group Size	small and medium
Materials	hats, scarves and caps
Duration	30 – 40 minutes

Sculpting can be used to illustrate and explore current concerns of members of the group. For example, people might be anxious about changes that have been announced or an individual may worry about an impending interview. Keep it general to start with and invite the group (in threes and fours) to sculpt a scene of wanting to buy something and the shop assistant not understanding them. Then role play the scene and see if the sculpt changes. Use this as a warm-up to sculpt a scene that one of the group members has offered such as being turned down for home leave. Create a sculpt of how he or she sees the beginning, middle and end of the interview. Invite people to comment on how a different outcome might have been achieved.

Variations

- If someone feels very threatened by someone else (friend, boss and so on), create a sculpt with one person standing much higher than the other; then see how it feels to change places (remember that a sculpt can always lead into words).

- Encourage people to think of a new situation that might cause anxiety: a new job, a holiday in a strange place and so on. Create a sculpt of the fears and then be able to talk about them together; then modify the sculpt.

- If there are going to be changes at the hospital or institution and so on, invite the whole group to create a sculpt of the good and less good things about the place now – and then a second sculpt of how they think it will be in the new place. Once we see something it becomes less scary. Then put together the good things from both places. Finally they can make a sculpt of the things they must say goodbye to.

5.9 Sculpting Polarities

Group Size	small and medium
Materials	none needed
Duration	20 minutes

You may have identified some feelings in the group and wish to explore these through sculpting. For example, in many groups there is an issue about trust – 'how far can I trust this person?' It may be personal trust or trust about confidentiality. In this situation you can create a diagonal sculpt with TRUST (I trust people very easily) at one end and MISTRUST (I don't trust people at all) at the other end. Invite people to place themselves on the diagonal in relation to their own feelings of trust and mistrust. Discuss where people would like to move along the line and the consequence of doing so.

Variations

- Encourage people to make a statement from where they are on the diagonal and where they would like to be.

- Invite people to take a quite different position and share how it feels.

- Invite one person to create the sculpt of where they see people.

5.10 Sculpting 'Then' and 'Now' Feelings

Group Size	small and medium
Materials	none needed
Duration	20 minutes

Bring the group together to have a discussion about 'how we see ourselves' and 'how others see us'. For example, people say things like: 'My father always thought me a pretty little girl but I still feel awkward and clumsy'. Then create the diagonal again and people take it in turns to stand on the 'line' where others see them and then where they see themselves. The ends of the line may change with individual people and can be a variation of, for example, overweight or just right; shy or confident; lonely or sociable. It is important that everyone 'hears' what people actually feel about themselves.

Variations

- Suggest to the group that people try someone else's perceptions of them and then share how it feels.

- Create the idea of 'this is how I feel now' and 'this is how I would like to feel'; then reflect in the group on what it would take to make that change.

- Instead of just standing on the line, suggest that people make the body posture and shape that goes with the feelings. Does it make a difference?

5.11 Sculpting with Chairs

Group Size	small and medium
Materials	chairs that are light to move
Duration	20 – 30 minutes

Some people get very stuck in the past or the present and this exercise can help people move on a little. You need three chairs and place them one behind the other. Explain to the group that the chairs represent the past, present and future. People then take it in turns to sit in the three chairs and speak about themselves: how they saw themselves five years ago, right now, today, and how they see themselves five years in the future. Allow enough time for everyone to try the chairs. Share a discussion of how people feel.

Variations

- If five years seems too long for some people you can do last week, today and next week.

- Encourage people to slowly extend the time – last month, now, next month; last year, now, next year.

- Suggest that people use the chairs to represent their childhood, themselves now, and themselves in later life.

5.12 Creating a Drama

Group Size	small and medium
Materials	pieces of cloth, hats, caps, props, old newspapers
Duration	30 minutes

When people have done plenty of warm-ups and movement, they will probably feel more confident about trying some drama. Keep your suggestions basic and simple with fairly conventional ideas. Start with giving everyone the opening line of a potential drama such as: 'Patty felt something was odd about this house and ...' or 'Gregory closed his suitcase and went downstairs, when ...'

Spend some time with people with ideas of how to start a drama. For example: How did Patty get there? Who is Patty? How old is she? Where is she? When does this happen? What is she doing? (the questions of how, what, where, when and why are all useful starters). After the exploration, people create their own drama and present it to the rest of the group.

Variations

- Think of some ending lines instead. For example: 'And that,' said grandmother, 'is the end of that', or 'Tune in next week to hear what Clarice did next'.

- Give everyone the same line, which has to occur somewhere in their drama, for example: 'Quickly,' hissed Janet, 'He is coming nearer', or 'If you say that again I am leaving,' snarled Bob.

- Cut out some headlines from a variety of newspapers and in small groups create a drama based on the headline.

5.13 Newspaper Stories

Group Size	small and medium
Materials	cloths, caps, hats, props and a variety of newspapers
Duration	30 – 40 minutes

You can either prepare this in advance or let members of the group choose: look through the newspapers and find short stories of events that have happened. It is not a good idea to use the more grisly or abusive reports. Choose short accounts of interesting court cases, unusual sightings, rescue by sea and land, for example. Let small groups choose which story they would like to dramatise and encourage them to ask the How?, What?... questions (see previous exercise). Dramatise and share the scene but try to discourage the groups from being competitive.

Variations

- Give everyone the same story and see the different interpretations of the same 'script'.

- Create a drama from an onlooker's point of view, for example the mother of the teenager who is rescued by helicopter.

- Imagine that the journalist actually made up the story because they were busy; create a drama about the journalist who wrote the piece.

5.14   Drama with Props

Group Size	small and medium
Materials	a varied collection of props: a walking stick, veil, newspaper, handbag, school case, pill-bottle, bunch of keys, dark glasses and anything else you can think of! It is not appropriate to include weapons or bottles of alcohol (unless you are running a specific group for people who are alcohol-dependent).
Duration	30 – 40 minutes

Every drama has significant props that help to move on the plot or that identify particular characters. Suggest that everyone chooses a prop and thinks about the character that would have such an object; how do they use it, where did it come from and so on? They can build the character and then introduce themselves to other members in the group.

Variations

- In small groups, people create a drama with three or four characters and share it with the others.

- Suggest that group members think of someone they know and an important object that person always carries (it could be a piece of jewellery that their grandmother always wears); each person tries to create their character and introduces them to the others.

- Invite everyone to create a play around some props that give the wrong information and really make sure the characters in the scene are very different.

5.15 Scenes to Dramatise – The Park Bench

Group Size	small and medium
Materials	cloths, hats, caps and props
Duration	20 minutes

Put three chairs together and make several park benches; if you have cloths to cover them, that is even better. Invite people to get into groups of three and give them the following characters: an old lady with a bag; a policeman; a professional woman with a briefcase. They can decide which character is sitting on the park bench and how they interact with the others. The person on the bench is the main character.

Variations

- What happens when all three characters are on the bench?

- Introduce the idea of rain or snow – what happens to the scene?

- Replace the policeman character with a newspaper seller.

5.16 Scenes to Dramatise –
The Old House

Group Size	small and medium
Materials	cloths, hats and so on; props
Duration	30 minutes

If you have a photograph of a spooky old house, it would be useful as a visual aid to this next drama; otherwise describe the house and encourage members of the group to embellish the details. It is derelict, gates hanging off the hinges, ivy growing around statues and so on. Suggest to the group that there are three people who are approaching the house. Invite the group, in threes, to decide who they are and what is their relationship and why are they going to this house. Improvise some ideas and then make a play.

Variations

- The people stand and listen, there is a sound coming from the house – what is it and does it make a difference?

- There is someone sitting in the garden, who is it and how do they handle it?

- Change the scene and decide that these three people actually live in this house – who are they and what is going on?

5.17   Scenes to Dramatise – The Demonstration

Group Size	small and medium
Materials	placard on stick, caps and scarves
Duration	30 minutes

Discuss with the group different sorts of demonstrations and street marches and how they feel about them. Would they ever go on a march? How would they feel if their photo was taken and put on the police files? Suggest people go into groups of four and choose different characters: one or two characters have placards supporting a cause; one person agrees with the march and the other person does not. Dramatise a meeting between them all and improvise the conversation.

Variations

- Create a demonstration that happened in Victorian times about the suffragettes and votes for women.

- Introduce one character who disagrees and believes that women should not have the vote or be educated or have careers.

- Create a freedom march for someone who has been imprisoned in a military regime; introduce a character who is against this person.

5.18   Scenes to Dramatise –
The Knock at the Door
(life and social skills)

Group Size	small and medium
Materials	none required
Duration	30 minutes

Create a group discussion about whether people should become involved in situations, that is, whether we trust our intuition and don't become involved or decide we are just being silly and over cautious. How can we take care of ourselves without letting it rule our lives? There could be many situations to explore that have happened in people's lives.

In pairs, one person is sitting watching television and someone knocks on the door; it is a familiar knock but it is dark outside. Improvise the possibilities of the situation.

Variations

- Suggest that there are two people in the house and one wants to open the door and the other does not.

- People decide what happens when the person knocking at the door sounds in great distress and asks for their help?

- If the person claims to be a legitimate caller: policeman or woman, meter-reader and so on, what do they do? The group improvise potential outcomes.

5.19 Scenes to Dramatise – Store Detective

(life and social skills)

Group Size	small and medium
Materials	none required
Duration	30 minutes

Create a discussion with the group about our human rights and what happens if we feel that people step over the borders. Are we OK about being searched? Do we mind if we are asked personal questions? Create a scene that involves three characters: a shop assistant, a store detective and a customer. The shop assistant thinks that the customer has been behaving suspiciously and has called the store detective. Make a drama about what happens and share the different outcomes.

Variations

- Add another character who is with the customer: mother or child? A couple?

- Decide that the customer thinks that the shop assistant is behaving strangely, what does she or he do?

- The shop assistant confides to the customer that the store detective is harassing her.

5.20 Scenes to Dramatise – The Airport Lounge
(life and social skills)

Group Size	small and medium
Materials	simple props, scarves
Duration	30 minutes

Create a group discussion about what we do when others ask us to do something that does not sound quite right. How do we feel about it? How do we handle it?

In pairs, create a scene at an airport; one character is a young woman who has saved up for a special holiday to Tunisia, the holiday of her dreams. As she is waiting in the departure lounge for a call for boarding, a man approaches her and suggests ...

Dramatise various scenes and share different endings.

Variations

- Suggest that the scene is changed to the security search and a suspicious package is found in someones luggage – what happens?

- Choose an alternative location in another country; suggest to the group that their wallet or bag has been stolen and someone comes up to them and offers to help – what happens next?

- Ask people to imagine they are sitting at a street table of a café in a foreign country; someone comes up to them and tries to persuade them to go with them to sight see or see a film or have dinner – how do they handle it? Make sure that they switch roles and also explore the dynamics for men and for women.

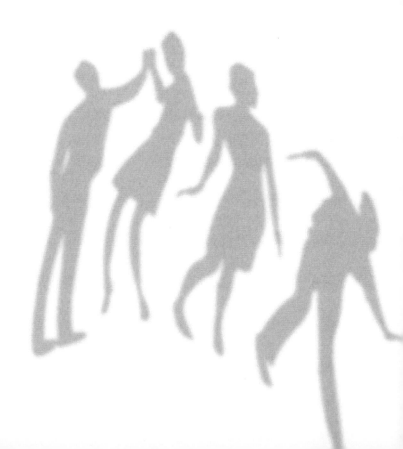

6 Stories and Documentaries

Most people like to listen to stories and many people enjoy telling stories, especially about themselves! With some individuals they will tell a repetitive story over and over again, often about a painful event from which they have not recovered. Stories in a sense are 'the fabric of society' as events and rules and customs are passed on from generation to generation. Sadly, much of this has been taken over by television where live interactive storytelling becomes a passive, spectator activity; many viewers feel quite intimidated by the skills of the stars telling children's stories. Some parents hand over the storytelling activities to CDs and DVDs rather than tell stories themselves.

This section is about different storytelling activities and can usefully be combined with activities in the following sections: Pictures and Images (pp95–116), Drama and Role Play (pp117–137) and Puppets and Masks (pp155–168).

I have included the idea of documentaries because for some people it is less scary than the idea of storytelling. Creating a documentary about a person or a place is something readily grasped by many people, as they see documentaries on television. However, all of it is storytelling in some shape or form and by encouraging it people will gain in confidence and improve their social skills. And it is important to remember that stories do not only have to be in words; we can tell stories through pictures or sounds or movements, or a combination of several media.

6.1   Basic Story Frameworks

Group Size	small
Materials	none needed
Duration	20 minutes

It would be useful if you can have a general discussion about stories and remind people that they are always telling stories: when they are waiting at the bus stop, talking to the doctor or e-mailing a friend. We do not always realise that we keep telling tales, even to ourselves!

Suggest to people that they sit in pairs and take it in turns to tell their partner the story of their journey to the group today. Whether they just walked down the corridor or whether they caught a bus to the centre, something will always have happened on the way.

Variations

- Invite people to tell the story from when they woke up this morning to now, to their partner or small group.

- Each person takes a special object or a photograph out of their bag or pocket and tells a story about it.

- Everyone tells their partner the story of the (top) clothes they are wearing.

6.2 When I Woke Up this Morning...

Group Size	small and medium
Materials	people sitting comfortably in a circle
Duration	up to 60 minutes depending on the size of the group

Invite everyone to settle into their chairs and take some deep breaths. Explain that so many of our day-to-day activities actually make stories, such as 'What happened on the bus' or 'What I saw in the park', but we don't always think about them as stories. Then suggest that everyone closes their eyes, or lowers their eyes if closing them is difficult, and thinks back to when they woke up this morning.

Encourage people to tell the story called 'When I work up this morning', using as many descriptive words as they can. For example, did they wake suddenly or slowly? Could they hear anything outside – positive sounds such as birds singing or negative ones such as road drills? Were there nice smells such as toast, and so on?

Discussion
Having shared the stories round the group, discuss similarities and differences.

Variations

- Invite people to tell the story of a dream they remembered when they woke up.

- Ask people to tell the story of everything they notice in their room when they sit up in bed.

- Encourage people to tell the story of a photograph or picture that they have hanging on their bedroom wall.

6.3   Storytelling Aids

Group Size	small
Materials	a large basket with a collection of different objects that can stimulate a story such as: anniversary card; lace handkerchief; brass door knocker; old family photograph; ceramic pot; peacock feather…
Duration	20 – 30 minutes

Invite everyone to sit in a circle and warm up into stories. Then pass the basket round and each person takes out an object that catches their eye. They hold it for a few moments and then tell a story about the object. Often people can hold an object with their eyes closed and become very inspired. The story is the right story, whatever it is and it does not have to be an accurate association with the object.

Variations

- Suggest to people that they take out an object with their eyes closed, so they choose it by touch.

- Have a basket that has just natural objects: stones, shell, bark…

- Fill the basket with a wide variety of old photos – easily found at car boot sales.

6.4   The Box in the Attic

Group Size	small
Materials	a small box or bag or attaché case with a collection of objects, such as: rosette, birthday card, key and small book of poetry
Duration	30 – 40 minutes

Place the container of objects in the middle of the circle and invite people to talk about whether they have any connections to each other. They were found in one container – who might they belong to? Why did they keep them?

In smaller groups, ask people to create the story that connects all these objects. Suggest that it is a romantic story.

Variations

- Change the thinking to the possibility of a mystery story.

- If it is a new group use fewer objects, maybe just two.

- Suggest to members of the group that they choose some objects.

6.5 The Cup in the Attic

Group Size	small
Materials	an award cup for gardening or embroidery or cookery; if you cannot acquire a cup, create a certificate and print it on old paper that looks like parchment. Pen, colours and paper
Duration	20 – 30 minutes

Encourage a discussion in the group about surprises that we find out about people: awards they received, achievements for skills we did not know they had. Sometimes it is members of our own family or close friends – sadly it can be after they have died and we discover things they have stored away.

Explore the cup (or certificate) and individually create a story about the person who it belonged to. What sort of person are they? Why did they keep it secret? Does it change your opinion of them?

Variations

- Invite people to imagine the cup or certificate belongs to a relative of theirs. How would that change how they feel about them?

- In twos or threes suggest that people create a fantastical story about the winner of the prize, and share it with the group.

- Encourage people to create a certificate for themselves for something they have done that was not recognised, then tell the group the story of their achievement.

6.6 Documentary about 'My Street'

Group Size	medium and large
Materials	pens and paper, prop microphones and cameras
Duration	30 – 40 minutes

Have a group discussion about documentaries: what sort do people like? Are they true or are they exaggerated? How are the cuts made when the final programme is made?

Suggest that people make groups of five and discuss making their own documentary about a famous street or the street where the hospital or day centre is situated. They can do interviews and take pictures and then show their documentaries to each other.
Set a time limit – maybe 10 minutes maximum.

Variations

- Allow people to do some research on their street project and bring back more information the following week.

- Allow the group to choose a theme for a documentary. Encourage them to keep it simple and short; people learn to prioritise and include the most important themes and facts.

- Suggest that people create a documentary about a special member of their family and include other members of the group in their play.

6.7 New Product Documentary

Group Size	small and medium
Materials	pens and paper; Blu Tack
Duration	20 – 30 minutes

Start a group discussion about promotion and advertising and how new products are sold. When is it impressive? What promotions do we remember? The music, the pictures, the colours and shapes?

In small groups think of a brand new product – think of all the things that would sell this product. How would group members advertise it? How would they make a symbol that will be remembered? Invite people to create a documentary about this new product and show it to the others.

Variations

- Think of a product that no one would ever buy; what story could group members tell to persuade people to buy it?

- Think about a popular type of product and invite people to create a story so that no one would buy it!

- Some products are never promoted and not really known – I wonder why? Think of something that faded away because it was not promoted. Encourage people to create a story that might change its fortunes.

6.8   Tall Stories

Group Size	small and medium
Materials	paper and pens
Duration	20 – 30 minutes

What do we mean by a 'tall story'? Tall stories originated in the 19th century when people would tell exaggerated tales that were not true in any sense; some people attribute Baron von Munchausen with their origin, stories were told that were wildly exaggerated. 'Tall talk' originated even earlier as contrasted with 'small talk', the former indulged in by men and the latter when women joined them!

In twos or threes create a 'tall story' in which everything is exaggerated. Think of a larger-than-life character who does wildly unlikely deeds or achieves stuff that dreams are made of! Encourage people to share their tall story in a serious way so that they don't laugh while they are telling it.

Variations

- Discuss what characters would not be larger than life – invite people to think of an unlikely hero character and create an 'anti tall story'.

- Encourage people to create a story where they are talking about themselves and wildly exaggerate things they have done.

- Think of the opposite – a character from a film or novel or television programme – who would never be a larger-than-life figure; invite people to tell a story that underplays this character and see whether they are still interesting even if they have not done great deeds.

6.9 Postcards for Stories

Group Size	small and medium
Materials	pens and paper, assorted postcards
Duration	20 minutes

Start the session with everyone sitting in a circle discussing postcards. Do people like receiving postcards? What is the most unusual postcard people have received? Do people send postcards themselves? How do they choose who to send them to?

Share a set of postcards that show holiday places; everyone chooses a card and with a partner tells a story about the place pictured. They can share whether their partner would have told a similar story or whether the postcard stimulates a different theme for them.

Variations

- Invite people to tell stories with a set of postcards of trees or flowers or rainbows.

- Find postcards that have traditional pictures and slogans and encourage people to tell stories.

- Choose old postcards that have messages on the back – think about who might have written the postcard and to whom; suggest the group create a story about these people.

6.10 The Dancing Camel

Group Size	small and medium
Materials	cloths and scarves
Duration	20 – 30 minutes

The following is an ancient story from Persia. Tell the story to the group and share their impressions. Allow everyone to have a copy of the story so that they can re-read it for themselves.

In ancient times merchants would travel along difficult and tiring routes in order to trade material, jewels and precious metals.
They would travel in groups, usually by camel and the paths were dangerous. Robbers would waylay travellers and steal their precious merchandise, which is why they travelled in groups.

One such group travelled along a narrow and difficult path: the way was rough and rocky and the sun high overhead. One of the merchants suddenly pointed out a lush and green valley to their left. Everyone looked down and saw a wonderful place with a river running through it and the leader of the group suggested that they all go down and rest for a while. Their camels slowly and steadily walked down a steep path into the valley and an extraordinary sight greeted them.

There under a tree was a young boy, a most beautiful boy, and he was dancing a wonderful dance. He was quite unaware of the merchants and continued his dance. The merchants watched in awe, all except one of them who scowled and said to them 'Are you not ashamed that you admire someone who is displaying their body in this way – it is offensive to god'.

At that point the man's camel threw him to the ground. His camel then began to dance and followed the movements and rhythms of the young boy.

The leader of the merchants said, 'You see, the camel is dancing? If the beasts of the field can dance to praise the lord, why shouldn't we?

© Sue Jennings, 2008

This story has a twist that we are not expecting – how does it make a point? What is the point?

Exploration of the Story

1   Invite everyone to draw or paint a picture of this story; create the atmosphere of the landscape and the colours.

2   In small groups re-create the story through movement.

3   Turn the story into a play with costumes: cloths and scarves.

4   Imagine that with the group of merchants is a young camel boy who looks after the animals when they have stops. Invite people to tell the story of the journey and the encounter with the dancing boy as seen through his eyes. They can share their stories with members of their group.

6.11 The Story of a Child of Fire

Group Size	small and medium
Materials	dressing up clothes, hats and caps
Duration	30 minutes

This is a story from the Pacific, near to Hawaii. It allows us to explore the many aspects of fire and its energy.

In a village near Hawaii lives a young girl who loves lighting fires. She loves the smell of the wood smoke, and the sound of the crackling twigs, and her eyes light up at the glowing embers and she can see all sorts of pictures and stories in the dancing flames. Soon the other children join her; they roast vegetables and dance round the fire singing songs.

The other parents come and visit the girl's mother to complain at the bad influence she is having on their children. And her mother has to say to her daughter, 'You are making our life very difficult here; so you have to stop lighting fires'. The girl finds this difficult but she does try. She goes for a long walk and reaches a huge field, far away from the village. 'Ideal for us' she thinks, and runs back to the village to tell the other children. They plan a picnic and go off for the day; they drag logs and branches to make a fire and cook their meal. They tell stories and sing songs and soon it is time to pack up. Just as they are putting out the fire, a man appears waving his arms and shouting. It is the farmer who owns the field and they all run as fast as they can back home. The farmer follows and starts knocking on the doors of the houses asking for the children who lit the fire in his field. The adults tell him to go to the girl's house, which he does, and he speaks very angrily to her mother.

Her mother talks to her again and says that this time is her last chance, otherwise she will have to leave home. The girl is really sorry and tries very hard to do other things instead. But she still longs for her magical fires and keeps wondering whether there is another place. She and just some of the children decide to go off for the day (the others were too scared of perhaps meeting another angry farmer). They walk for a very long way and find a place on the other side of the forest on a piece of rough ground that does not appear to belong to anybody. They light their fire and sing and dance, but most especially they tell stories. They cook vegetables which were especially sweet that day. Little did they know that this might be the last time they had this adventure. Or maybe they did know and were determined to make it the best they had done. They go home happily and are not aware that the smoke is drifting upwards across the top of the forest towards the village. People open their windows and sniff: hmmm – woodsmoke – that girl. Her mother is waiting for her and tells her that she has had her last chance and that she must leave. The girl packs a bundle, ties it to a stick, puts it on her shoulder and walks away.

She looks after herself, cooking her food as she goes, and soon she comes to the seashore. She lights a fire from driftwood and sits gazing out to sea. A water sprite called Nimusha says she does not like the girl lighting fires and she is stronger than she is. The girl challenges her to a trial of strength. Nimusha creates a tidal wave and the girl turns it into a twenty-foot high jet of steam. She enjoys making explosions under the sea and starts to create volcanoes, and makes her own island. She creates the biggest explosion she has ever done and makes the volcano her home. She rides her chariot across the flames, laughing as she goes, and the young men of the village create games of prowess on the rim. The older people of the village decide to protect themselves and they make offerings of white sweet-smelling hibiscus flowers and throw them into the crater.

Meanwhile the girl is becoming calmer and is less angry and spends more time curled up asleep at the edge of the volcano having wonderful fiery dreams.

And now, if you are visiting there, you may see a little old woman with grey hair and a tattered red shawl. And she may just come to you and ask you for matches and a candle. The old woman keeps her fire and, if pressed, may even tell you a story or two. And her eyes will still light up at the memories of her fiery life.

This story is important because it expresses the cultural values from the society where it originated. Although we may want to modify certain stories that have inappropriate violence, we must stay true to the essence of the story.

© Sue Jennings, 2006

Exploration of the Story

1   Discuss this story – especially the reactions of all the adults towards this child.

2   Tell this story in groups with movement – spend some time exploring the scene between fire and water.

3   What do people think the child's mother is thinking and feeling? Create a story with her as the main character.

4   Create a play of this story in small groups and share it with other groups.

5   Invite people to create their own story based on the other elements: earth, water and air. Illustrate them and read them out to the group.

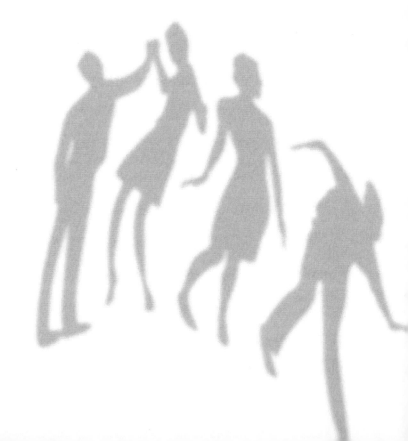

7 Puppets and Masks

Several of the previous sections have techniques that can be developed with both puppets and masks. There are also many ideas for making your own puppets in *Creative Puppetry with Children & Adults* (Jennings, 2008) so I am not dealing with puppet-making in this section.

There are superb hand puppets for working with all groups of any age and often the most listless and non-communicative individuals will come alive when they see or hold a puppet. Puppets should never be imposed on people because some people need time to get used to playing with puppets again as they may think it is a childish activity. In my own resources I have the following as a basic minimum:

- large puppets that can sit on the knee with moving mouth and arms (several skin colours and hair styles)

- sleeve puppets that are soft to the touch: domestic pets (cats and rabbits) and wild animals (wolves, foxes, harp seals, elephants)

- finger puppets that tell tales (gingerbread men, grannies, Red Riding Hood set).

When you are using masks you need to take care that people do not feel stifled or get 'lost' in their mask. My guideline is to use handheld masks made from decorated papers plates and glued to a stick for most mask work, otherwise masks that only cover the eyes which can be highly decorated with beads, feathers and so on (*see Creative Play and Drama with Adults at Risk* Jennings, 2005b). I only use full face masks for training courses.

With suitable caution puppets and masks can enhance your groupwork and stimulate people's creativity.

7.1 Playing in the Orchestra

Group Size	medium and large
Materials	some easily held sticks (dowel rod in 18" (46cm) lengths is suitable but always check for splinters); CD player, CDs of orchestral music
Duration	15 minutes

This activity can be used as a means of leading into other stories and drama and it can be used as a warm-up in its own right for puppet work Explain to the group that the sticks are to be used for a very specific purpose and that there must be no hurting of others. Invite everyone to be a conductor using their stick while you put orchestral music on the CD. Allow people to have fun with this first and exaggerate the conducting and use whatever gestures they like. Then suggest that everyone can choose a musical instrument and play as if they are in the orchestra and take it in turns to conduct. This gets people used to using their bodies to express ideas in varied and interesting ways.

Variations

- Suggest to people that they can make small groups of similar instruments: 'the strings', 'the brass', 'the wind', 'the percussion' and so on; then they play together within the bigger orchestra. Sometimes the conductor will indicate they have a solo while the other musicians wait.

- Invite everyone to imagine that they are a musical instrument – not that they are playing one but that they are one – how would they move? People can guess what instrument everybody is.

- If you feel the group trust each other, invite people to make pairs (I suggest men with men and women with women); one person is the musician and one person is the musical instrument; encourage people to be inventive in terms of how they use their bodies. Now you have another orchestra and people are using each other like puppets.

7.2 The Puppet Orchestra

Group Size	medium and large
Materials	CD player and orchestral and jazz CDs
Duration	15 minutes

This will really test people's ingenuity and you would not use this exercise with a very new or inexperienced group. Invite people to make groups of four or five and suggest that they create a puppet orchestra. Some people will be the instruments, others will be *puppets* playing the instruments, and one person a conductor.
It takes a lot of trust and imagination, not to mention coordination, but it can be a really fun exercise to do. Share the activities with each other.

Variations

- Invite people to imagine they are playing in a music festival and each group is entering.

- Try the same exercise but using jazz music instead.

- Repeat it again but have a singer in the group instead of a conductor.

7.3 Tell Me a Story, Please

Group Size	small and medium
Materials	large puppets with speaking mouths
Duration	20 minutes

People will need time to get used to working with these puppets and you may not have enough for everyone to have one each. So this will be a lesson in turn taking! Invite people to make groups of three or four; one person has the puppet and tells a story to the group. You can suggest a well-known fairy story to get people started and members of the group can prompt if people get stuck. Remind people that the puppet is a storyteller rather than a character in the story.

Variations

- As people become more confident they can experiment with telling a personal story through the puppet or telling some invented gossip or a news item that has been reported.

7.4   Creating a Puppet Play

Group Size	small and medium
Materials	small hand or sleeve puppets of animal characters or people (try to avoid puppets from TV series or people will rely on the stories and not invent their own).
Duration	20 – 30 minutes

It is important to have enough puppets for everyone to have one each and some left over so that people have a choice. Initially, invite group members to choose a puppet and have some fun with it, experimenting with how to move it and creating expressions. Then in groups of three or four, people can tell a story that involves all the puppets and one person is the narrator (this guards against people thinking they have to put on silly voices).

Variations

- Suggest to the group that they think of a situation that needs discussing but they discuss it through the puppets – this often gives people more confidence to say their point of view; share the debate with the others.

- Invite people to choose a puppet as a leader in a crisis and then choose other puppets to be in the scene and create a play.

- Introduce the idea of a puppet play that can teach others about 'life and social skills'. Suggest to the small groups that they create a situation where others can learn 'appropriate behaviour'.

7.5 Broomstick Puppets and Masks (1)

Group Size	small and medium
Materials	wooden broomsticks, paper plates, fabric for cutting and draping, old hats, PVA glue, scissors, old wool
Duration	30 – 40 minutes

You will need careful panning so that there is time both for making the mask or puppet and then for using it: you may decide to do it over two sessions. Check the wooden broomsticks for splinters. If they are too big for some people to hold then use dowel rod. People create a character by draping and gluing pieces of fabric on to the stick; create a face by gluing pieces of felt onto a paper plate; add a hat or hair from the wool and so on. Once they have made the character they can think about who it is and give it a name. People can introduce their new companion as they sit in small groups.

Variations

- Invite people to walk around the room with their broomstick puppet and introduce it to other people; they need to find a way to greet each other.

- Suggest to people that they create groups of characters that might know each other and encourage their puppets to talk to each other.

- Change it to just random groups of people who do not know each other and find ways to communicate.

7.6 Broomstick Puppets and Masks (2)

Group Size	small and medium
Materials	broomstick puppets as in the previous exercise; rhythmic music CDs, CD player; basic props such as sunglasses, binoculars, handbag
Duration	20 – 30 minutes

Introduce to the group the idea that instead of having a large puppet on a stick, they now have a mask that they hold in front of themselves. People will speak in the first person and introduce themselves, whereas with the puppets they would have used the third person and said 'This is ....' Once they have introduced themselves to the whole group they can then form smaller groups and create a scene to enact about a topic of their own choosing. Remember that everyone is now the character themselves and using the stick puppet as a mask.

Variations

- Invite people to add a prop to their character such as sunglasses or a pen; see what difference it makes to the character.

- Suggest that they tell a story in the first person to a partner, through the medium of the puppet/mask.

- In threes, introduce the idea that there is a conflict between two of the puppet characters and the third person helps to sort it out.

7.7 More Personal Exploration

Group Size	small
Materials	large and small puppets of all kinds
Duration	20 – 30 minutes

Invite people in the group to choose a puppet to express a feeling: for example, they might choose the wolf to be angry or the harp seal to be shy. Allow time for different puppets and feelings to be experimented with before asking everyone to choose one puppet to focus on. In groups of two or three encourage people to use their puppets to express feelings and say why: 'I am very angry because...' The other puppets can respond and agree or disagree or make suggestions. Make sure everyone has time to express what they are feeling.

Variations

- Invite people to use the puppets to express something more personal about themselves; not an in-depth disclosure but something they feel worried or anxious about; the puppets can then discuss the issue and make suggestions.

- The same as above, but instead of discussing it the puppets make a puppet play to find a solution.

- Suggest that people choose a puppet to express their dream of life – what would they really like to do; share it in the small group and comment in a positive way.

7.8　Masks of Opposite Feelings

Group Size	small
Materials	paper plates, scissors and crayons, stapler, wool, small fabric scraps
Duration	20 – 40 minutes

Invite people to make two masks using the paper plates and crayons: one mask to show a positive feeling and the other to show an unhelpful feeling. Give people enough time to cut out eyes and mouth if they wish and maybe attach some hair or fabric. However, set a limit of 20 minutes unless you want to make masks in one session and then use them in the next session.

If this is a group of no more than six people then they can sit in the circle and introduce themselves through the two masks, holding one up at a time. Suggest they say the unhelpful feeling first and then the positive one afterwards. Compare similarities and differences.

Variations

- Explore the same exercise but suggest that people both express the feeling and say *when* and *where* they feel it (not why).

- In pairs suggest that the masks can talk to each other – one positive talking one with one unhelpful one.

- Create a group of similar masks and suggest that people add words and movements to express the feeling. See if the different groups can have contrasting expressions.

7.9 The Story of the Bored Young Prince

Group Size	medium and large
Materials	broomstick puppets or paper plate masks, fine elastic; lots of fabric in long swathes and rainbow coloured if you can or create rainbow materials by painting plain fabric with multi-coloured paints; paper and paints, crayons
Duration	30 – 40 minutes over several sessions

Give everyone a copy of the story and encourage them to read it through; then go round the circle and everyone reads a few lines (they can opt out and gesture the next person if they wish).

The Story of the Bored Young Prince

In ancient times there was a young prince who spent most of his time being very bored with life. He seemed to have everything that he wanted and he was still not satisfied and the members of his staff were at their wits' end to know what the best thing was to do.

His faithful counsellor with his long grey beard kept trying to find new and interesting things for the prince but to no avail. One day the prince said that the counsellor had to find something new to interest him or there would be trouble. The counsellor went to the kitchens and spoke to the cooks and said that they had to produce something very special by the following morning and after some protest they agreed. He then went to talk to the carpenters and said that they must produce something new and different by the next morning or there would be trouble. They were shocked at the short space of time but the counsellor persuaded them to be ready at the palace gates the next morning. Finally, he went to see the musicians and asked them to compose new music for the prince and they said it was impossible in such a short space of time. The counsellor said that their very lives could depend on it and that they must try. So the musicians said that they would stay up all night and do their best.

Wearily the counsellor went home to bed and dozed very fitfully until dawn. He looked out of his window in the turret and there were the cooks and the carpenters and the musicians all lined up outside the palace gates. They went in through the great studded doors into the prince's presence where he was lounging on a couch. The cooks presented their food and he immediately shouted at them and said it was boring; the carpenters carried in the most beautiful carved box you have ever seen inlaid with mother-of-pearl and he chased them out of the room. The musicians sang their new song for the prince and he shouted at them to disappear as they were making a dreadful sound. Everyone slunk home in disappointment and the prince called the counsellor to him.

He said that he had to find something new or there would be very great trouble and he was giving him one last chance. The counsellor was very fearful because the prince was SO angry and feared he might lose his head. This time the counsellor went to see the clowns and the poets and the astronomers and pleaded with them all to create something new for the prince by the following morning. He emphasised that they would all be in great trouble otherwise. And the next morning all of them were there with special gifts for the prince. Again, the prince became angry and said that the clowns were not funny and the poets not poetic and when the astronomers had found a new star and named it after him, he exploded and shouted that he did not want to be a small star amongst millions!

The counsellor became very fearful and pleaded to the prince for one last chance. He went to his turret and sat in his chair looking out over the city. He felt at his wits' end and the tears streamed down his face and trickled through his long grey beard. Then as he looked through his tears he began to form an idea that perhaps could work. He wiped his eyes and went out into the dark night and went to the workshop of the silk weavers. He explained his idea and they were very intrigued. But when the counsellor said that it had to be completed by the very next morning they were aghast.
The weavers said that it was quite impossible but the counsellor silenced them and said that everyone's lives depended on it.

He went home with a heavy heart and did not sleep very much. In the morning he looked out of his window and saw that the silk weavers were indeed there at the gates. He went down and joined them as they were ushered into the presence of the prince. He was looking particularly bored as they entered, carrying a large roll of material.

They unfurled the silk on the floor in front of the prince and explained that it was rainbow silk, woven especially for the prince. There was complete silence as they all waited for his response and the counsellor was extremely nervous.

The prince got up slowly and picked up the end of the silk and wrapped it round his shoulders and walked round the room. Then he did a little dance, swirling the silk as he went, and it shimmered and shone in the beams of light coming through the windows.

He then stood still and looked at everybody and said that he had treated them all most cruelly and had rejected all the good things they had done for him. He was truly sorry for behaving so badly and would try to make amends. By way of showing how sorry he was he decreed that everyone in the city could now wear rainbow silk, which they did, most joyously.

And the counsellor remembered that he had seen rainbow colours through his tears when he was so distressed in his room the night before. The rainbow colours of his tears had inspired the weavers to make rainbow silk.

And that was how the prince and all the people of his city became joyous now that they were wearing their rainbow coloured silk.

© Sue Jennings, 2009
(Adapted from an ancient Persian tale)

Exploring the Story

This is a longer story than the ones we have used so far and really makes a whole project to explore over several weeks so the following exercises do not have to be hurried. Slowly the group can build up the whole story for people then to enact as a whole.

1   Invite people to talk about the story first and to share which character they would like to explore and why.

2   The groups of crafts people can be varied and others introduced if you wish. Invite everyone to choose a craft and then work at it in small groups; emphasise the skilled movements that people use.

3   Then add words: what do cooks (no celebrity chefs perlease!) and carpenters talk about when they are working? Who is more senior? Who is learning the trade? Encourage people to bring it

to life rather than just doing the task. Slowly they will find they are developing the characters rather than just being a carpenter.

4 Invite people to create a picture of the particular thing they are making.

5 In small groups explore what might have happened to the prince's parents. Why has the counsellor to take all this responsibility? What has made the prince as objectionable as he is?

6 Why is the silk so significant? Did the counsellor know that this was important? How do people feel about him crying and then getting inspiration?

7 Create a 'day in the life of the court' with everyone going about their business – maybe there is a market where people sell their wares?

8 Invite people to create broomstick characters and use them like masks to speak through (remind them that when they are playing the character, carrying the broomstick will limit their movement) – or they can create a 'half-mask' with the paper plate so that it only covers half their face and attach it to their head with fine elastic.

9 Create a group picture of the rainbow silk on fabric or paper.

10 When the groups feel ready suggest they create a play based on the whole story. Maybe they will decide to have a narrator.

11 Share and process the play in the following session – what people enjoyed and what they would like to change BUT make sure that everyone 'breathes in' their achievements.

8 Cool Downs and Closures

It is really important that you structure your groups in such a way that there is ample time for closure work. It is easy to get carried away by the enthusiasm of group members or to forget the time and then people will leave the group in a stimulated or even anxious or hyperactive state. We all need to cool down after any type of mental or physical activity and have a period of calm. It does not need to be deep relaxation as that could put people to sleep but it does need to enable people to leave the group calmly and as individuals. This especially applies if they have been doing intense groupwork together.

There are relaxation exercises already described in previous sections so I will not repeat them here. They can be used as part of a 'cool down' process at the end of your group.

However, I will include some other 'de-roling' techniques (1-14, pp170–171) that are also important when group members have been playing different characters and wearing masks.

It is important to remember that some people can get so involved in their masks that they won't take them off. You need to be firm and give a count-down for everyone to remove their masks.

Also, I think you need to be careful about instigating group discussions as a matter of course at the end of the groups. It can feel a bit like school when everyone went on a school trip and then had to write about it. I will often say, 'Is there anything anyone would like to say?' or 'Do people want to share anything about this session?' People then feel they have a choice and some people like to stay with their own thoughts and feelings while they are processing them.

1. De-roling: Invite people to stretch and yawn and allow the role to slip away from them. Vigorously shake or jump and feel their body changing back into their own body again.

2. Suggest that people walk round the room while they shake off the role and make any sound that comes to mind.

3. After physically de-roling they say one at a time: 'I am no longer … (the name of the character) but I am … (their own name).

4. As themselves discuss in the group what people learned from playing the role – what did they find out about the character?

5. Invite people to stand in a circle and to close their eyes; ask them to picture the character they have played and the gestures and body movements – suggest that they let go of the gestures and body movements and now picture themselves with their own gestures. The people can open their eyes and walk round the room as themselves.

6. Repeat the exercise as above but with their eyes open, invite people to make the exaggerated movement of their character before letting it go.

7. People can then make their own movements very exaggerated before owning them again.

8. invite people to walk round the room and shout their own name as loudly as they can and then as quietly as they can.

9. Using a chair: invite people to place a chair in front of them and to imagine that their role is sitting on the chair – in their posture and wearing the clothes and props. Then they see the character as separate from themselves and say goodbye to it and feel they can walk away.

10 Invite people to place the mask of the puppet on the chair and follow the exercise as described above.

11 Another way is for the person to sit in the chair as their character and then to get up and walk away as themselves.

12 Suggest that people imagine their character is sitting in the chair – they go up to the chair and invite them to dance – they dance with their chair around the room and then say goodbye!

13 People stand anywhere in the room and slowly retrace the steps that their character took and then move into walking as themselves.

14 Invite people to sit in the circle and go through the whole sequence in their mind and then let it go.

15 Everyone stands in the circle holding hands, thinking about something significant that they will take away from this group. When they open their eyes they acknowledge everyone in the circle.

16 Think of the story of the *Wizard of Oz*: group members share whether they are taking away courage, or a brain or some feelings, or that they know their way home!

17 In the group circle, people say one thing that they appreciate about each member of the group.

18 Encourage people to keep a diary or journal about their journey through the group: make time at the closure to write down thoughts and feelings.

19 Invite people to draw a symbol in their diary to represent how they are feeling at the end of the group.

20 If it is the last group of all, spend more time on processing what has been discovered and everyone's appreciation of the contribution of other people.

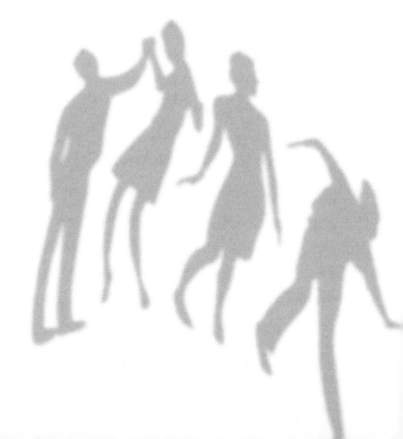

End Piece

By writing this new edition of *Creative Drama in Groupwork* I am moved to share yet again my own convictions about this type of work. Creative drama is not just a way of keeping people occupied or a collection of techniques, it is a process that we can encourage in order to keep our groups more healthy and alert.

In these days of yet more television and ipod, it is important to remember that face-to-face human interaction and opportunities to create and share together, all contribute to human well-being and happiness.

It is sad that stress and anxiety amongst our 'clients' and also the staff in hospitals, prisons, day centres and special schools is increasing, despite new approaches to therapy, workers, charters and health and safety.

Creativity for all of us needs to be in place both at work and home so that we can all reach our fullest potential. Let's learn to play again and the rest will follow. As I said at the beginning – go slay the dragon and bring back the treasure!

Sue Jennings
Glastonbury 2010

Resources

There are many universities and colleges offering qualifying courses in the Arts Therapies as well as short introductory courses and summer schools. Please consult the following websites for up-to-date information. For overseas training and projects please email: rowancentre@gmail.com

Training courses leading to a Dance-Movement Therapy MA

Dance-Voice Bristol

Goldsmiths College (University of London)

Queen Margaret University

University of Derby

University of Roehampton

University of Worcester

Professional Associations

The Association for Dance-Movement Therapy UK, (ADMTUK)
32 Meadfoot Lane , Torquay TQ1 2BW

admin@admt.org.uk   www.admtuk.org.uk

Birmingham Centre for Arts Therapies
Stratford House, Stratford Place, Highgate, Birmingham B12 0HT

mail@bcat.fsbusiness.co.uk   www.bcat.info

Training courses leading to a Dramatherapy MA

Anglia Ruskin University

University of Roehampton

Central School Sesame
(London)

University of Worcester
(approved training in Exeter)

University of Derby

Professional Associations

The British Association of Dramatherapists
Waverley, Battledown Approach, Cheltenham,
Gloucestershire GL52 6RE

enquiries@badth.org.uk   www.badth.org.uk

BadthResearch@yahoogroups.com

The Sesame Institute
27 Blackfriars Road, London SE1 8NY

info@sesame-institute.org   www.sesame-institute.org

Training courses leading to an Art Therapy MA

Goldsmiths College
(University of London)

University of Edinburgh

University of Hertfordshire

University of Belfast

University of Roehampton

University of Derby

University of Sheffield

Professional Associations

The British Association of Art Therapists (BAAT)
Mary Ward House, 5 Tavistock Place, London WC1H 9SN

www.baat.org

Training courses leading to a Music Therapy MA

Anglia Ruskin University

Nordoff-Robbins School, London and Manchester

Queen Margaret University, Edinburgh

The Guildhall School of Music and Drama, London

University of Roehampton

University of the West of England, Bristol

Professional Associations

The Association for Professional Music Therapists (APMT)
(now incorporates The British Society of Music Therapy)
24–27 White Lion Street, London N1 9PD
APMToffice@aol.com

Music as Therapy
The Co-op Centre, 11 Mowll Street, London SW9 6BG
alexiaquin@musicastherapy.org   http://www.quin.eclipse.co.uk

Training courses leading to a Play Therapy MA

University of Canterbury

University of Glamorgan

University of Roehampton

Professional Associations

British Association of Play Therapists
1 Beacon Mews, South Road, Weybridge, Surrey KT13 9DZ
info@bapt.uk.com   www.bapt.uk.com

Play Therapy UK
The Coach House, Belmont Road, Uckfield, East Sussex TN22 1BP
ptukorg@aol.com   www.playtherapy.org.uk

Other websites

www.actionwork.com

www.psychodrama.org.uk

www.londoncentreforpsychodrama.org

www.creativepsychotherapy.info

www.rowancentre.net

www.dramatherapy.net

www.suejennings.com

www.projectwolf.co.uk

Bibliography

Anderson-Warren, 1997, *Creative Groupwork with Elderly People,* Speechmark, Bracknell.

Boal A, 1992, *Games for Actors and Non-Actors,* Routledge, London.

Cattanach A, (ed) 2002, *The Story So Far: Play Therapy Narratives,* Jessica Kingsley, London.

Chabukswar A, 2003, *'Birth of a Story'* Prompt BADTh Summer

Chesner A, 1998, *Groupwork with Learning Disabilities,* Speechmark, Bracknell.

Crimmens P, 2004, *Storymaking and Creative Groupwork with Older People,* Jessica Kingsley, London.

Crimmens P, 2006, *Drama Therapy and Storymaking in Special Education,* Jessica Kingsley, London.

Gersie A & King N, 1991, *Storymaking in Education and Therapy,* Jessica Kingsley, London.

Hickson A, 1997, *The Groupwork Manual,* Speechmark, Bracknell.

Jennings S, 1983, *'Models of Practice in Drama Therapy' in Journal of Drama Therapy, Vol. 7, No. 1,* BADTh, Cheltenham.

Jennings S, 1997, *Playtherapy with Children: A Practitioner's Guide,* Blackwell Science, Oxford.

Jennings S, 1998, *Introduction to Dramatherapy: Ariadne's Ball of Thread,* Jessica Kingsley, London.

Jennings S, 1999, I*ntroduction to Developmental Playtherapy: Playing for Health,* Jessica Kingsley, London.

Jennings S, 2000, *Brigid: Fertility, Creativity and Healing,* Rowan Studio, Wells.

Jennings S, 2001, *Inanna: Journey into Darkness and Light*, Rowan Studio, Wells.

Jennings S, 2003, *'EPR – A Model for Dramatic Play',* in Play Words, April/May.

Jennings S, 2004a, *Creative Storytelling with Children at Risk,* Speechmark, Bicester.

Jennings S, 2004b, *Goddesses: Ancient Wisdom in Times of Change,* Hay House, London and San Francisco.

Jennings S, 2005a, *Creative Storytelling with Adults at Risk,* Speechmark, Bicester.

Jennings S, 2005b, *Creative Play and Drama with Adults at Risk,* Speechmark, Bicester.

Jennings S, 2005c, *Creative Play with Children at Risk,* Speechmark, Bicester.

Jennings S, 2006, *'An exploration of creative ageing and social theatre', Journal of Nursing and Residential Care, 8 (1), pp29–31*

Jennings S, 2008, *Creative Puppetry with Children & Adults,* Speechmark, Bicester.

Jennings S (ed), 2009, *Dramatherapy and Social Theatre, Necessary Dialogues,* Routledge, London

Jennings S, 2010a, *101 Themed Story Starters,* Hinton House, Milton Keynes.

Jennings S, 2010b, *Healthy Attachments and Neuro-Dramatic-Play,* Jessica Kingsley, London

Jennings S & Hickson A, 2002, *'Pause for Thought: Action or Stillness with Young People',* in *Communicating with Children and Adolescents,* eds Bannister A & Huntingdon A, Jessica Kingsley, London.

Jennings S & Minde A, 1993, *Art Therapy and Dramatherapy: Masks of the Soul,* Jessica Kingsley, London

Johnston K, 1981, *Impro: Improvisation for the Theatre,* Methuen, London.

Lahad M, 2000, *Creative Supervision,* Jessica Kingsley, London.

Landy R J, 1989, *Dramatherapy Concepts and Practice,* Charles C Thomas, Illinois.

Levy G, 2005, *112 Acting Games,* Meriwether, Colorado Springs.

Pitruzella S, 2004, *Introduction to Dramatherapy: Person and Threshold,* Routledge, Hove.

Sherborne V, 2001, *Developmental Movement for Children,* Worth Reading, London

Slade P, 1995, *Child Play: Its Importance for Human Development* Jessica Kingsley, London.

Warren B, 1993, *Using the Creative Arts in Therapy,* Routledge, Hove.